Wings of Light
Feet of Clay

On the Nature of Healing

Gretchen Weger Snell, PhD

Copyright © 2021 Gretchen Weger Snell

All rights reserved. No part of this book may be reproduced or utilized in any form or by any means, electronic or mechanical including photocopying, recording, or by any information storage and retrieval system, without permission in writing from the author.

All rights reserved.

ISBN: 9798710265192

DEDICATION

A note of Gratitude to all the teachers and visionaries who had the courage to follow a different path; to my clients, students, friends and family who continue to teach and inspire me daily; to those who have helped who make this work possible; to the bright children who are changing the world for the positive; and for the healing of the Earth and all her inhabitants.

*And for my son,
who is the greatest gift life has ever given me.*

DISCLAIMER:

The information in this book is not intended to replace professional medical treatment. Consultation and continual treatment with the medical doctors advised. The tools of philosophies presented in this work are not intended to diagnose or treat disease, rather to present a scientifically credible proposal to bridge both conventional and traditional healthcare therapies.

PREFACE

This work is dedicated to all those who refuse to stand powerless in the face of illness.

To those who intuitively know that healing involves reclaiming health as a multidimensional experience.

To those who open their minds to look objectively at the alternatives that are undeniably causing healing and doing so in clearly observable, measureable and provable means.

Here lies a different path; may you walk it in gentleness and beauty.

TABLE OF CONTENTS

	Preface	v
1	Introduction	1
2	A Different Path	15
3	Tree Bark	25
4	A Quantum Leap in Perception	35
5	The Vital Force of Healing	45
6	Symptoms as a Roadmap to Healing	53
7	The Elements of the Wheel	67
8	The Healing Power of Man's Energy	89
9	A Quantum Blueprint for Healing	112
10	Closing	142
	Bibliography	150
	About the Author	157

INTRODUCTION

The winding, arduous path to this sacred grove requires two things - effort and persistence. The view is breath-taking. This vision creates pause, full stop, with attention arrested into the fullness of the present moment. Gradually and almost imperceptibly, every fiber and knot tied up with the past, and what pulls forward toward the future releases. Body and soul fills with wonder and gratitude on the deep breath that grounds being into just this present moment. Released into the true nature of our human being rather than our programmed mode of doing. This right here, the ever-present "now" where all true power and possibility are present, is the gift of the trip. Silence. Majesty. In a slice of time beside still waters, painted sky, gentle breeze brushing through the leaves, the incessant grip of reality slips to reveal a deeper reality.

In this place outside time, the sage waits. In his wrinkled leather face of the old sage, age was a mystery. Every crevice embodied a path of trial and wisdom worn *irrevocably into the fabric of a lifetime. The intensity of his eyes deep sparkling pools of vitality, and compassion, yet piercing into your soul, which remains fixed in their grasp. The smell of burning sage, cedar and lavender permeates the air. Each herb holding unique medicine released when burned, to purify and create sacred space.*

"So, what is it that you seek?'" he asks from under furrowed brow. His eyes sparkle as he studies the young healer.

"Healing", the young healer answers.

"Are you unwell?" queries the sage.

"No. I feel fine. It's just…something…missing….", the voice trails off. "I guess I was seeking your guidance. What is it that is missing, that I am missing? Where do I go from here?"

"Why do you ask questions from me when the answers lie within you?" he replies with a piercing stare. "Why would you seek outside for others to determine your destiny? You are in control of the choices that determine your life on this earth path."

The healer hesitates, thinking, "Those who seek my help...they are sick. They take medicines and get better, but the cycle repeats. They never seem to get well, vibrant, thriving, you know, with that exuberant spark to be alive."

"Ah," says the sage, "what you seek is wholeness. To help heal in the true meaning of the word: 'to make whole'. That, my young friend, requires a radical revision in perspective and approach."

The sage continues, "Man has never been strictly physical. To focus on the material realm is temporary. Correcting physical manifestations only addresses results, the cause of which remain hidden in the interior. Man is multi-dimensional, thus healing therapies must attend to many levels. That is what brings wholeness and healing."

"But if all I see is the end result...how do I access these inner, multi-dimensional realms of which you speak?" asks the healer.

"Come," beckons the sage, "I will show you. But first, you must open your mind to the idea that just perhaps, it is the patient that will heal you!'

In the late evening hours, the healer contemplates the experiences of the journey thus far. Barely perceptible yet, on a level beyond the five senses, the gentle pulse of transformation stirs. Old forms that no longer serve loosen; old structures crumble to make way for powerful new growth. From this ancient place of power, a new journey beyond expectation had been initiated.

A space to stop, breathe and stand, centered in the present moment. That elusive, present moment when we hop off the proverbial hamster wheel and become human beings rather than human doings. For a few moments, we set aside the cares and worries that perpetually distract our minds from the inner power of our sacred selves. The sage used that term - our sacred selves - in conjunction with wholeness.

The dictionary defines sacred as, *"The power understood to be at the core of existence and to have a transformative effect on our lives and destinies"*. The sacred is deep and abiding, within each and every one of us, yet dulled by the incessant noise of daily life. The old sage emphasized stillness. Each step taken on the healing path requires time spent in the stillness of the present moment. Modern civilization finds it difficult to stand still and be fully present. Yet cultivating this ability promotes transformative power in life. From our center, being in present time is where truly profound and lasting changes take place. Infinite possibilities surround us from where we have the power of choice. Our potential and our power for transformation lie within the ability to cultivate this still point, to find our sacred center of balance.

Curious, notes the healer that, "the power understood to be at the core of existence" has been neatly excised from the current practice of conventional medicine. No longer understood to be at the core, in its wake we find a mechanistic model of linear cause and effect of man as a machine where broken parts can be replaced. Mechanical growth and repair is programmed and predicted by DNA. Perhaps a radical revision in the linear perspective and approach is indeed precisely what is required.

What if the current, conventional Western medical approach is only a fraction of the truth? Man has never been strictly physical, said the sage. Have we narrowed our perspective of nature into one accepted mechanical model while turning a blind eye to the wisdom of the ancients? Is it possible that there are layers of information, of the subtle energy of man which we have yet to acknowledge, let alone explore? And what if that energy contained the very information that we need regarding the roadblocks to obtaining full, vibrant, unstoppable potential?

After all the training, clinical experience and countless hours of searching, of one thing the healer was certain: the modern-day physicist and the ancient sages were essentially saying the same thing. The fundamental nature of matter is not matter at all; matter is essentially energy. Discoveries in the field of quantum mechanics proved that underneath what we know as matter, the subatomic level operates according to very different principles. At the most fundamental level, matter (particles) gives way to patterns of energy. The basic building blocks of matter, the particles – atoms, electrons, protons, and quarks - can only be defined in terms of motion, vibration, or spin. The manifestation of matter is determined by underlying forces of which we are only beginning to understand. And these forces, as of yet, can only be observed through their interaction with matter (particles). Life is at once unpredictable and inexplicable.

The healer contemplates the shifting sands around the bedrock of material science. Groundbreaking research in the field of medicine demonstrates that regulation and communication within living organisms can no longer be adequately explained through strictly chemical means. Likewise, communication occur faster than can be explained by electrical nerve transmission. Research indicates that electromagnetic frequencies attenuate cellular receptors facilitating communication within living organisms. Moreover, it has been demonstrated that coherent energy fields guide the growth and regeneration of cells. These energy fields possess intelligence and a language of their own, comprising a system that communicates information according to the principles of quantum mechanics. These fields communicate instantaneously, to every level of the body. More importantly, they can be directed to positively influence our healing process. But, because we cannot see them or touch them, they are dismissed. Perhaps we are dismissing vital critical information that could provide a very different roadmap to healing?

For the young healer, the time spent in this ancient place of power emphasizes the estrangement of man from Nature. Humans are seen as separate from and "above" natural world, a world viewed as mechanical parts. In the time of Hippocrates, and today in indigenous cultures, energy or spirit was viewed as subsisting in all forms of life. This force protected the natural world, and nature supported man. When mankind is separate from and exalted above the natural world, it becomes too easy to claim dominance and exploit natural resources.

Earlier, the sage inquired as to why the healer would embark on this journey. The healer was searching for more natural ways of healing; perhaps the ancient ways were far more powerful than given credit. Then there were the inexplicable cases of spontaneous remission. How was it that simple herbs and homeopathic remedies produced such deep and lasting results? Even more perplexing were the sessions in which spontaneous moments of profound realization for a client produced instantaneous shifts in energy, which promoted lasting, positive results. Nothing in the current model of molecular chemistry could account for this. The sage reached over and touched the healer on the forehead. At once, a door was opened to a memory where questions lay unanswered. The sage listened intently as the experience unfolded.

It was one of those moments where time stops and everything shifts. The healer's father received the diagnosis of cancer. The kind that was inoperable and fatal. Questions formed that were nonstop and, unmercifully, met without answer. How did this happen, and why wasn't it found earlier? Every day the healer sat watching an IV drip "medicine" into his arm, talking him through his hallucinations, and holding him when he was too weak to stand. Many months prior to this diagnosis, it was apparent that something was not right. In conversations with his father's physician, the healer discussed this perplexing situation. Father would develop an acute illness, then recover, only for this cycle to continue, but he never seemed to get well. He never seemed to regain that spark of vitality that made him, well, him. His doctor replied that he fully understood what was being asked, but he was afraid that modern medicine could not answer these questions. Anyone who has witnessed the progression of illness in a loved one has watched as that elusive vitality weakens over time.

"Continue," the sage encouraged. "What did you learn?"

"My father never did walk out of that hospital room. But I learned a great many things from that experience," the healer remarked. "I knew that somewhere we were missing key pieces of information, and that there had to be a different way, maybe even a better way."

Perhaps one of the most pivotal points of learning is that our material model of disease is outmoded and in need of revision. We do not "catch" a disease. Like health, disease is built, through decision and action. Disease symptoms represent the body's attempt to regain equilibrium. If we can learn to read these symptoms in that light, they could provide a personal roadmap to recovery.

"Your society has a saying," quipped the sage. "'Those who spend their health gaining wealth, later often spend that wealth regaining health.' I think it would be more prudent to say, 'If you build your health while building your wealth, you can enjoy your health while enjoying your wealth.'"

****

Every day we are doing one of two things: we are either taking steps to build health, or doing things to tear it down. Health starts with a decision, and the decision is which one of these paths you want to take. Examine your current state of health now and decide where you want to be in a year from now, five years from now. If your goal is vibrant health, then success will be determined by taking even small steps to produce those results. Nourish yourself daily - physically, mentally, emotionally and spiritually - and you will achieve amazing results. It is never too late to start and there is always room for improvement. Time is a precious treasure; it is something that you cannot bargain to gain back. What you decide today, and in this moment, will determine where you arrive tomorrow.

The condition of your mindset creates your reality. The condition of your body determines your ability to achieve your goals. And, the condition of your *energy* body determines the capacity to create both. Yet most of us have had scarcely any education regarding the hidden wisdom and extraordinary healing power of the energy body. That very topic is the focus of this work.

I have been blessed with the opportunity to assist numerous people on their healing journey by practicing and teaching the art of healing with natural medicine. It has been my passion and my hope to raise awareness of the incredible power of natural medicine. That natural medicine is both safe and effective, providing an alternate path to those who still are searching, and to enlighten those who may be unaware of their innate capacity to heal. To challenge the misperception that illness means we are broken and in need of repair. To no longer accept that there is no other way.

We can learn to read the language of our inner wisdom by considering symptoms as a roadmap to healing. However, this requires a new set of tools and a quantum leap in perception. We can then use this valuable information to direct our energy and positively influence our evolution, healing and spiritual growth to achieve our best life possible for ourselves and by extension, our community and our world.

WINGS OF LIGHT, FEET OF CLAY

CHAPTER 2

A DIFFERENT PATH

It was probably one of the most serious skin conditions I had yet seen. Truth be told, my initial reaction was to doubt my capacity to help. When little Adam arrived with his mother, his skin was so irritated it was literally raw over most of his body. Adam had been diagnosed with eczema. Different practitioners had prescribed various ointments from which he received very little relief or skin healing. My heart went out to them both, realizing that crying was the only way to communicate his pain and discomfort. I knew there had to be a different way, perhaps a better way not to solely provide relief but to promote healing. Something was off balance and I was confident that if corrected, his condition would improve.

Adam's eczema seemed to intensify when his mother had ceased breastfeeding and tried various infant formulas to supplement feeding. Additionally, a technologically advanced, non-conventional analysis uncovered an allergy. Adam's mother agreed to implement a therapy that consisted of feeding Adam goat's milk, in combination with taking several homeopathic remedies. This allowed for the readjustment of the microbes in the gastrointestinal tract as well as addressing the genetic weakness in the skin. Within the first month of the regimen his skin was about fifty percent healed and he was eating and gaining weight. With this progress, different homeopathic and herbal remedies were administered. After three months, the eczema had resolved almost completely except for a patch on the back of his neck and his knees. Pleased with his progress, his mother told me she had referred a relative for a consultation whose child, Daniel, was having digestive issues.

Daniel was three years old and had been having "loose stool" ever since his hospital stay to treat a Rotavirus infection within his first year of life. "I just can not bring myself to put him through that kind of intensive drug treatment again," his mother told me. Also, that they could offer nothing else like the herbal medicines her parents and grandparents had used in their home country. I assured her at that particular time the drug therapy probably saved his life. However, after the acute crisis had passed, a referral to a practitioner trained in the use of natural medicine to balance and replenish his body would have served to aid the healing process. While it is never to late to start and improvement is always possible, we would begin that process now. Since antibiotics are indiscriminant in killing both harmful and beneficial bacteria, the imbalance in the microflora of Daniel's gastrointestinal tract needed to be replenished with probiotics. His depleted body was nourished with key nutrients and trace minerals, and homeopathic remedies were implemented to return the body to homeostasis.

Improvement was very slow the first month. Daniel's mother was concerned that her son spoke very few words for a three year old. After an analysis of progress, new homeopathic remedies were administered. When they arrived for the third visit, his mother was smiling and happy to report that Daniel's bowel movements were normalized and that progress was being made in potty training. More surprising, Daniel walked up to me and spoke to me in complete sentences. I was shocked. To witness the power of this medicine to restore whole health was truly amazing.

And, as I was learning, this type of medicine is a well-kept secret; considered a type of voodoo medicine where amazing results are often discounted as placebo. How can the results of these events be reduced to a placebo effect in children of these ages? It would be erroneous to conclude that the transformation was purely coincidental; that the healing of the body had no bearing on the rapid change in Daniel's mental development. These stories fall outside the current framework, and fall through the cracks of the conventional medical system, yet demonstrate the potential healing power of natural medicine.

Take one more example of a different nature. Michael had been plagued with bedwetting his entire life (he was 19 years old). This negatively affected many aspects of his life including time with friends and even prevented him from college life that entailed roommates. Most of the credit for Michael's healing was due to his mothers unwavering devotion and absolute refusal to believe that there was no answer for her son. She was sure that there was no anatomical defect, nor psychological trauma that could account for his issue.

In his mother's words, Michael had been a trooper, willingly allowing her to drag him to every type of therapy (conventional and alternative) under the sun. She appeared in my office still hopeful for answers; Michael, with guarded optimism. Through a combination of advanced technology and classical homeopathy, Michael "healed" within a few months.

Advanced, non-invasive testing and analysis revealed a disruption of energy in his hypothalamus. One of the functions of the hypothalamus is to regulate sleep. His mother stated that Michael slept so soundly a bomb could explode and he would not wake up. This energetic imbalance in the hypothalamus was disrupting the signals that should have informed him to awaken, that the bladder needed to be emptied.

Using homeopathic and herbal medicines to alleviate the impedance, his condition was soon much improved. The incidences had been reduced to once or twice a week. Following the principles of classical homeopathy, an energetic predisposition was likely contributing to the problem. After a month using a different homeopathic remedy, the condition had been rectified. It has been years, and he still is free. Michael subsequently attended college and is married to someone with whom he has had the courage to share his story.

These cases demonstrate that if our ultimate goal is healing, then expansion of our current practices to include therapies that fall outside the realm of conventional medicine must be included, in order to address the whole person. To do so, we must address a few stumbling blocks.

First, in our Western mindset there is a lack of awareness and proper education regarding natural medicine. This leads to a second block, which is fear: fear that these therapies are neither safe nor effective. And third, that results from natural medicines are often not immediate.

This perspective can leave us in a very disempowered state. What we need is a change in perspective, a perspective where we can be empowered to direct and influence our own healing. After many years of seeking education from disparate healing systems and successful practitioners, I have learned that these stumbling blocks can be resolved. Comprehensive systems of natural healing do exist and can be taught to anyone open to learn. The remedy for that fear is proper education from reliable, trustworthy sources. An enormous amount of credible, scientific, clinically proven evidence exists proving that natural medicines can produce phenomenal healing results. And, although results may take a little longer, the payoff over-delivers.

I want to share a secret. We have the power to affect our health to a far greater capacity than we have been led to believe. We are born with a system of communication containing innate wisdom to continually maintain and build health. This system can be directed to positively influence your healing trajectory. This energy-based system communicates instantaneously, globally and cohesively to maintain and build health. Until recently, this system had been largely ignored by conventional medicine.

However, that is about to change. We are proving that we have the power to change the trajectory and affect our healing through the wisdom of the lost language of energy. This work presents an inception point for the necessity of integrating the energy bodies of man to create a comprehensive system of healing.

The knowledge of this inextricable link between the physical and energy bodies is the very basis of the healing systems of both ancient and indigenous cultures around the world today. Understanding the nature of the energy body and its effects on the physical body has allowed cultures to survive and heal since the dawn of humanity. If natural therapies did not work, mankind would be a distant memory in the history of life on earth.

Only recently has the existence of the energy body gained consideration as a legitimate field of study in the health sciences. Discoveries in quantum physics as well as progress in unveiling the energy portion of man are challenging the prevailing theories of conventional Western medicine. This compels an adaptation of our approach to include electromagnetic fields and subtle energies as vital for healthy communication and healing. This will necessitate a shift in our materialistic approach in medicine to include the discoveries of quantum physics, which redefine frequency as the basis of our physical reality. It will require a re-vision in order to integrate the wisdom of the traditional forms of natural medicine with the technological advances of conventional Western medicine.

For this revision, the existing fracture that separates conventional Western medicine from natural medicine must be healed. The thesis of one system need not be the antithesis of the other. Rather, we need a synthesis that incorporates both, without dilution of the strength of either approach. The prevailing mindset of the seeming polarity perpetuates a non-necessary division. What is lacking is an understanding of the wisdom of the lost language of the vital body that serves as a bridge to connect both sides. To truly support the health and healing of humanity, a comprehensive system of medicine must be revised to be inclusive of the bioenergy system of mankind. We must create a synthesis of therapies that address the whole of the human condition, to encompass the sacred nature of our multidimensional being.

****

For the sake of clarity, the term "conventional medicine" will be used to define our current practice and teachings of modern medicine in the hospitals and universities of the Western world, inclusive of all advanced technology, research and pharmaceutical interventions. This approach is based on Newtonian or classical physics. The term "natural medicine" will refer to alternative approaches such as herbal and homeopathic medicines, energy and vibrational therapies and acupuncture. This philosophy incorporates the principles of quantum physics and consciousness

CHAPTER 3

TREE BARK

The old sage sent the young healer out on retreat: a quest of sorts before resuming instructions. "How can you possibly know where you're headed if you don't know where you've been?" asked the sage. "You're like that leaf floating in the stream, without any care or direction. How can you shape your goals or influence the path of your direction if you don't acknowledge the progress that led you to this point?"

"There is a saying among the natives of the Americas, 'That which you refuse to confront continues to walk with you.' Until you acknowledge your accomplishments, then face your demons, the patterns you have created will continue to unconsciously carve your destiny."

For the next week, the old man sent the healer away for solitude. First, the healer was instructed to recall and acknowledge professional accomplishments made thus far in practice. This would provide fortitude to take the next step - to briefly note any unresolved matters and any demons that continued to haunt the path of personal progress. Those, the old man said would be addressed at the teaching of the Wheel. Finally, the old sage required the healer to examine the field of medicine and healing. To recognize the accomplishments of those who carved the path, the giants on whose shoulders we stand. And from that point, seek to uncover any the shortfalls that are awaiting fresh ideas or radical approaches for possible resolutions.

****

For those who have experienced the power of natural medicine, similar questions invariably arise. Why haven't we heard of this earlier? Why are we using synthetic drugs with side effects when we could use natural remedies? And perhaps most importantly, why are conventional and natural medical system antagonistic with one another? Many of those who have dedicated their lives to the study of conventional medicine wonder why, with all our advances in modern medicine, is it even necessary to revive the discussion of seemingly archaic ideas of herbs, homeopathy and the vital energy body?

Advances in conventional medicine over the past century, both pharmaceutical and technological, have saved incalculable lives. Many of us and our loved ones are alive due to these advances in conventional medicine. However, the same cannot be said for chronic diseases, which continue to escalate in modern times. The Centers for Disease Control's own website states that about half of all adults have one or more chronic health conditions; one in four adults has two or more chronic health conditions. And that, "chronic diseases and conditions such as heart disease, stroke, cancer, diabetes, obesity, and arthritis are among the most common, costly, and preventable of all health problems." The United States ranks low for indicators such as infant mortality and life expectancy.

The pressing need to bridge this gap is best exemplified by a story relayed by a client. He went to his internist to monitor his chronic condition. After several questions, the client received a lecture regarding his choice to use natural therapies along with conventional medicine. Indignantly, the doctor stated that the two medicines absolutely cannot work together, and that if his patient thought that tree bark was going to heal him he was obviously deranged. Curious that the doctor specifically referenced tree bark since Samuel Hahnemann, the father of homeopathy, serendipitously stumbled upon both a treatment for malaria *and* the basis of homeopathic medicine using the quinine-rich bark of a Cinchona tree.

When new information collides with established theories, we are forced to make a decision regarding how to assimilate this new information. Do we cast aside the information as an anomaly, or face the disconcerting fact that our current perceived constructs of reality must be shifted to accommodate new truths?

Discoveries that oppose prevailing scientific theories are often initially rejected. Prior to the information discovered by Copernicus, we were certain of earth's position as the center of the universe. Galileo was imprisoned when he challenged the prevailing theories of Copernicus. Alfred Wegener challenged the fact that the earth beneath our feet is indeed not "solid", rather the continents slowly drift around the earth, morphing over time. Although Pythagoras postulated the notion of a spherical earth, the idea was resisted until Magellan proved that ships would not fall over the edge of the earth.

Resistance to change can be a formidable adversary, especially when observations and undisputable evidence directly oppose accepted scientific "fact". This resistance has restrained and even denigrated evidence of the validity of natural medicine and the efficacy of its modalities. Quite often facts have been discarded and relegated to the files of unknown phenomenon in an effort to avoid the discomfort and uncertainty of reconstructing the foundation of our current medical system. Science, by its core principles, continually seeks to challenge any accepted theory of life and our natural world by attempting to disprove the very theory it just proposed. The true student of science (and by extension, medicine) must stand ready to revise their understandings and beliefs independent of emotional attachment, even if it threatens to redefine the very system within which they work.

The divergence in philosophical approaches to healing depends on how we define health. That definition determines how we build a system of medicine to achieve and maintain it. The conventional definition of health is, "Physical and mental well-being; freedom from disease, pain or defect; normalcy of physical and mental functions, the state of being free from illness or injury ". This defines health as the absence of something else. Health is much more than merely the absence of disease, pain, defect or injury.

Our practice of peering down the microscope to examine finer and finer unseen parts has given medical research a myopic perspective that somewhere "down there" we will find the answers to life and health. Philosopher and mathematician René Descartes introduced this perspective, termed Reductionism, to Western philosophy in the early 1600's. This view postulates that man and the natural world can be understood if first broken into basic elemental parts; then by reassembling these components we can recreate the whole.

Reductionism extricated spirit from the physical form, leaving a partial and wholly inadequate perspective to explain life and the natural world. The vital energy or spirit was relegated to the mythical ethers and considered no longer necessary for the evolution of life. From this window, life becomes a meaningless set of circumstances impinging on the physical body, which continually adjusts to the environment and is completely under the jurisdiction of the programming from the DNA in cells. It also perpetuates our illusion of external control in that chemical deficiencies can be synthetically repaired and worn out parts can be replaced.

A further divergence in philosophical approaches to health care occurred in the 1800's. The prevailing medical philosophy at that time held that diseases were cause by miasma - a polluted environment, vapors from organic rotting matter, and conditions of poor hygiene. The idea of miasma was supplanted by a new theory known as germ theory, which proposed the idea that certain diseases are cause by microorganisms.

Germ theory established microbes as the foundation and causative agents of disease. Thus if the microbe could be eradicated, it would eliminate disease. This germ theory was supported by the advent of antibiotics (truly miracle drugs at the time), which saved countless lives in the face of epidemics and acute diseases. The prevailing theory of the day viewing environmental conditions as the cause of disease was discounted, replaced by the notion that an identifiable agent could now be found and eradicated. The modern approach was set for heroic interventions that attack and destroy the enemy without much consideration as to the groundwork that allowed for the disease development, with little attention paid to the overall condition of the body (the "battlefield") after the treatments were applied.

Eradicating disease through the application of a single treatment, a type of linear medicine, while effective in the face of epidemics falls short of an explanation for the true cause of chronic disease and ill health. Microbes cannot be the sole causative agents, or the diseases they are treating would strike all health care workers in emergency rooms and hospitals. And some individuals who have been vaccinated against a certain germ still end up contracting the disease. Certain geographical areas are affected by disease and others not. Some family members develop influenza and others not - while being exposed to the same microbes. The explanations and treatment for acute diseases do not translate into healing chronic diseases.

Research laboratories are in perpetual search for the one substance (virus, bacteria, fungus, gene) that produces the disease (effect). Lab results, diagnostic tests and blood work often cite a static condition, a snapshot in time. While providing valuable information, this describes a limited perspective. This current model streamlines the process allowing for quick diagnosis and prescription of therapy. Once diagnosed, it may be possible to slow the process with synthetic drugs, surgery or radiation, but implies that the process will continue in that one direction, a direction of degradation. A linear approach certainly simplifies the process, fostering an illusion of possessing the capacity to exert control over the process. While effective in acute situations and emergencies, this linear approach however, falls short of providing curative treatment in chronic conditions.

We have strayed far from the perspective of Hippocrates where, "It's far more important to know what type of person the disease has than what type of disease has the person." In contrast to our current conventional system, the focus of natural medicine is on the health of the individual rather than the state of disease; on what causes and rebuilds health. Health is viewed as the sum total of a multifaceted and dynamic process. Disruption on any level can affect multiple systems and lead to disease. A myriad of factors impact the body and affect multiple processes on both physical and energetic levels. This explains the basic divergence in the two medical philosophies. Natural medicine practitioners observe and attempt to locate the source of the disruption, and then intervene to support regenerative outcomes. Positive results can be realized through combinations of traditional medicines, energy therapies and cutting-edge technologies. And even occasionally, with tree bark.

CHAPTER 4

A QUANTUM LEAP IN PERCEPTION

The discoveries of Albert Einstein and Max Planck regarding energy and matter have yet to be fully incorporated into our current system of medicine. The principles of quantum mechanics have shed new light on our understanding of the material world, and we find that the principles of classical physics break down in the subatomic world. Matter appears to defy what science, and by extension medicine, knows as "fact." Rather than the linear, predictive, continuous models, we find a fascinating new world.

That the concept of energy was an integral part of healing is evidenced by the use of the term "medicine" in contrast to modern day. The word medicine has been pared down to being synonymous with a substance that is ingested to treat disease or pain, and the science of treating and curing disease. To the ancients and the indigenous people today, the word medicine implied an inherent power, a force unique to and a part of every object in the natural world. They understood that energy and matter are bound together and intricately related long before this was "scientifically proven" by Einstein and Planck.

As discussed previously, both pharmaceutical and technological advances in conventional medicine have saved numerous lives. However, many questions remain unanswered. Genes and germs fail to provide a complete explanation for disease. Identical twins do not always contract the same disease. Professionals working in emergency rooms are not all afflicted with the current epidemic plaguing their patients. For those with open minds, it is increasingly apparent that the materialist, mechanistic view of Western science is incapable of providing all the answers.

Any new data discovered regarding the electromagnetic and subtle energy body is not intended to disparage or discount any form or conventional therapies.

Rather, the emerging information enhances and deepens our understanding of life and healing. Without question, it is absolutely essential to maintain the physical body with the utmost care. Without the physical, there is no ground for the energy to manifest. Restoration and maintenance through nourishment with whole, organic foods and herbs is of fundamental importance for optimal health. Numerous books have been written regarding this subject. Entire lines of nutraceuticals and herbal supplements are continually being developed to support life-sustaining chemistry. My students are encouraged to remember the story of *The Three Little Pigs* and decide for themselves if they would like to build their "houses" of straw, sticks or bricks.

Yet we are learning that we are so much more than simply matter. Humanity is awakening to the incredible power we have to influence our own healing. We all have the capacity to change the trajectory from disease to health. When working with natural medicine, we are working with natural law. Nature holds all things in balance. We merely need to shore up deficiencies and remove impedances, then let the vital body restore homeostasis for healing. This means deficiencies and impedances in the energy realms as well as the physical. Already, we are aware that mental and emotional stressors (energy) can have a profound effect on the progression or regression of disease. The relationship between stress and disease has been well established thanks to the work of Dr. Hans Selye in the 1950's. Additionally, for the past twenty-five years the Institute of HeartMath has been conducting substantial research documenting how implementing techniques for stress reduction profoundly improves a wide variety of health issues. That the essential nature of attending to deficiencies and impedances in the energy body is likewise essential for health has been proven for millennia by the systems of Chinese acupuncture and the Native American system of the "rivers of light".

A new model of medicine is emerging that is integrative in approach and provides fresh perspectives. This model includes the subtle energy bodies and electromagnetic fields of man. The principles of quantum physics help redefine the conventional model with a new understanding of disease and the healing process. In this emerging paradigm, information is communicated instantaneously through the body's energy fields. Much work has been done to illustrate the theory that these coherent energy fields regulate the chemical and molecular processes of the body. A thorough analysis of this subject can be found in Gerber's comprehensive book, *Vibrational Medicine*. Numerous reactions simply cannot be explained sufficiently through the old model of classical physics. A current working model proposes that energetic changes in the environment are transduced through the energy body, and then communicated to the physical body. Light energy flows through the acupuncture meridian network; DNA communicates through light particles known as biophotons. This energy is distributed through the body via a microscopic neural network into every cell of the body.

The mechanistic world, one that conforms solely to the laws of classical physics, is an outdated model. Our scope has been restricted to what is detectable through the five senses. Except for a few tests, electroencephalogram and electrocardiogram, acknowledgement of the energy body is virtually non-existent. The model of linear cause and effect allows for predicted outcomes that can be manipulated by physical and chemical controls. When a part wears out, it can be removed or replaced; chemical imbalances are synthetically addressed. The unknown nature of energetic variables places a mysterious force in the equations removing that illusion of control. Add to this the most recent discoveries of the nature of consciousness and healing, and we wander into unknown territory. To maintain that illusion of control, the current conventional system is at a loss as to where to place energetic information.

Only recently has the existence of the energy body gained consideration as a legitimate field of study in scientific and medical studies. Acupuncture has earned some acceptance and is even practiced in some hospitals since the existence of the body's meridian system has been *scientifically verified* with a super quantum interface device (SQUID). Interestingly, entire cultures and systems of natural medicine have thrived without the need for previous confirmation from a SQUID. Research has proven that much communication occurs faster than can be explained by electrical nerve transmission. According to the work of Fritz Popp, we learn that all living cells produce and communicate through biophotons (light energy) at high-speed transmission. Scientific evidence supports the theory that information transfer occurs energetically through the biophotons in a coherent field of light. (Popp, Chwirot,

Roeland and Van Wijk).

Many of these processes, which remain mysterious, find possible explanation within the principles of quantum physics: in particular, the discovered principles of non-locality, discontinuity and entanglement.

The quantum principle of non-locality describes an instantaneous transfer of information or energy without the exchange of signals though space-time that is required by classical physics. The quantum model postulates that both the subtle energy and the physical body are quantum fields existing as waveforms of potential. As both are "quantum correlated" objects, a change or disturbance in one will manifest in the other simultaneously, without the local exchange of signals (Drs. Goswami and Drouin).

Next is the observance of the principle of discontinuity. In contrast to classical physics, changes in a quantum system go through a "leap" from one energy state to another without going through linear, connected steps. When a change occurs on any level, the possibility waves "collapse" into a new state discontinuously to a localized particle all at once. This quantum leap helps to explain sudden changes, "leaps" in healing, and spontaneous healing.

The third principle is that of entanglement. Entanglement underscores the novel idea that both practitioner and client are intricately engaged in the healing process. This process, known as a tangled hierarchy, is both unique and individualized - in contrast to the current conventional model.

Innovative research supports the idea of the living organism being a quantum system that operates according to quantum principles. In her book, *The Rainbow and the Worm; The Physics of Organisms*, Mae Wan Ho describes living organisms as "quantum coherent exhibiting the properties of quantum superposition (unlimited possibilities in potential), delocation, inseparability and non-local interactions" (Ho, 2008, p. 280). In accordance with Erwin

Schrödinger's discovery of quantum entanglement, Ho states that, "A quantum coherent system has neither space nor time, so the collapse of one part is instantaneous communicated to other parts, regardless of how great a distance separates the two" (ibid).

Quantum theory has demonstrated our unified wholeness, and our energetic basis. The material model provides only one perspective. The error in thinking occurs in accepting the corollary to this material model, which implies "to the exclusion of all else". Conventional therapies work with physiological changes in tissue structure and function. However, cutting edge research demonstrates that changes occur in the energy fields prior to these physiological manifestations. Various balancing mechanisms and feedback systems are in place to compensate for disequilibrium and attempt to reestablish homeostasis. Perhaps most intriguing, as will be discussed later, advances in technology allow us to observe and monitor these changes so that progress in the healing process can be assessed.

WINGS OF LIGHT, FEET OF CLAY

CHAPTER 5

THE VITAL FORCE OF HEALING

By now, the old sage had started referring to the young healer as Bendith. It was an ancient Celtic word meaning "strength, health and success achieved through one's own merits". Bendith may need that strength today meeting the new sage. If rumors were true, she did not suffer fools lightly.

Tall, cool, with a faint blue cast to her aura, Arwyn appears to glide into the grove. "Come closer," she beckons. "I'm not so formidable as you've been told. What I do require is your full attention and a stout heart. For what I shall speak of alters the foundation of your material medicine."

"Tell me what you know of the vital force and

homeopathy," Arwyn asks.

Bendith details the background. Over two hundred years ago, Samuel Hahnemann, the father of Homeopathic Medicine, introduced a radical new theory based on natural law. This form of natural medicine was successfully practiced prior to the advent of germ theory.

"And Paracelsus before him", she interrupts, "though he was dismissed. Even though our ancient forms of healing are based on this understanding of energy. The notion of a vital force has been an integral part of the medical philosophies and sacred texts of cultures around the globe."

She continues, "Vital force is known by different names in each culture. Chi in China, Prana in India, Ki in Japan, Spirit by Native Americans, Pneuma by the ancient Greeks, Num by the Kalahari, and Mana by the people of Hawaii."

Bendith pipes in, "Our modern scientists call it Orgone, Ether, Bioplasmic Energy or the Universal Life Force."

"Yes", she answers coolly, "leave it to modern man to think they discovered something new. As far back as the 3rd Century BC, the Greek anatomist Galen held the belief that vital spirits were necessary for life. The concept of vital life force energy was at the heart of the healing process. Even Hippocrates recognized the existence of the hidden forces that are the healers of disease. A description of life and health without this understanding presents the basis for many misconceptions."

In a melancholy tone, she continues: "When the vital force that permeates all life was ripped from its roots, nature and the material realm lost its sacred, inviolable quality. This established a new paradigm of 'power over' versus 'power within', leaving the material realm devoid of innate wisdom and intuition of the energy body to be dominated by the mind and external authorities."

Bendith understands that this "vital force" was a central tenet in homeopathic philosophy. Hahnemann postulated that this vital energy animates the body and strives continually for balance, or homeostasis. It is proposed that the vital force enters the material body at the time of conception and exits at death.

"Now pay close attention", she directs, "as this will answer some of your questions. This vital force pervades the entire organism, maintaining a state of working equilibrium. Therefore, a disruption of any nature in one area of the body disorders the vital force, producing an effect in the entire organism. An imbalance results and the vital force attempts to regain equilibrium. These attempts represent functional changes that are occurring as the result of disruptions in the realm of force, the realm of physics, prior to manifestations of any tissue changes. This is the true meaning of 'Holistic Medicine' rather than what it represents in the common vernacular as the use of vitamins and herbs instead of drugs."

She continues to explain that symptoms are to be recognized as the body's primary reactions to regain balance: a change in energy precedes a change in chemistry. This reaction is the expression of a functional imbalance that is occurring in the energy realm, the realm of force.

And with a stern look she adds, "Without a comprehension of the role of the vital force in the healing process, you are missing the boat. Without it, disease becomes the enemy, an immaterial substance that must be expelled or annihilated. However, symptoms are to be read, addressed and supported - not to be suppressed and attacked. When these symptoms are suppressed, the cause of the imbalance is neither addressed nor removed. Rather it is driven deeper into the body into more vital organs and processes."

From this Bendith realizes why previous teachers stressed that suppression of fevers and skin rashes could cause other issues down the line. Medicines could be given for symptomatic relief, but that would not necessarily address the underlying cause. Of course, training dictated that at times it may be necessary to intervene with a drug to save a life, or temporarily take over the function of a failing organ until the crisis has passed. However, after the crisis has passed, natural interventions to rebuild the body and halt recurrences are rarely addressed.

"Our scientists have a tough time with this", Bendith remarks. "If it's not measurable, or observable by the five senses, it's dismissed as pseudo science."

"Well", she demands, "I guess scientists need to decide if they seek truth or not. Is it not the very nature of science to continually challenge accepted theories by attempting to disprove the very theory it just proposed? Even if new theories threaten to redefine the very system within which they work, regardless of beliefs or emotional attachment? Is science now based on consensus? Sounds more like religion."

Bendith decides no comment was best at this juncture.

The sage explains that the Vital Force itself is not visible to the naked eye; however its effects on the body can be observed. A disturbance in the vital force becomes evident manifesting as symptoms. However, these symptoms are the effects of disease; the cause being a disturbance in the vital force.

If the vital force were capable of doing the healing alone there would be no disease effects in the body. Rather, its job is to return the body to a state of balance so the body can heal itself. From a point of homeostasis, the body contains all the wisdom necessary to build health. Free from symptoms, pain or disease, the mind - endowed with the gift of sound reasoning - can utilize the human body to achieve its higher purpose of existence in this life, its goals, dreams and mission.

Arwyn ends with a final warning. "Although the vital force is energy, spirit-like, it would be a mistake to equate it with the Soul or Spirit of the sacred texts and religious philosophy. The vital force is the energy that animates the body, maintaining harmonious operation. It regulates and balances the bodily processes of constructive and destructive metabolism. When this balance is disrupted, it predisposes the body toward a disease state. This vital force is an innate energy. It does not make conscious decisions. However, in its absence, internal *processes become strictly catabolic, returning the body to the base minerals of which it is composed."*

With a flourish and a bow, Arwyn leaves Bendith to digest the lessons. Ultimately, medicines should be aimed to support and strengthen the power of this internal healing force, to promote health and the healing process. In the words of Hahnemann, "The highest ideal of therapy is to restore health rapidly, gently, permanently; to remove and destroy the whole of disease in the shortest, surest, least harmful way, according to clearly comprehensible principles."

CHAPTER 6

SYMPTOMS AS A ROADMAP TO HEALING

She was slight of frame and tiny in stature, yet one piercing look from our 90 year-old instructor would cause us to freeze like a deer in headlights. It was a true privilege to learn from her. She had studied natural healing therapies and medicine from every continent on the globe: some recognizable, others bizarre and inexplicable. Yet her most fascinating aspect was her disregard and defiance of the disease title pronounced upon her at 22 years of age. Now in her 90's, she stood in front of the class, stuck out a rock-steady arm and asked us defiantly; "Do you see any Parkinson's here? When they made that incompetent diagnosis at 22, I told them they could take their Parkinson's and shove it! Of course, that set me on this path to take care of myself as I wasn't about to take anyone else's opinion." That day she gave us a crystal clear view of the unwavering commitment and drive it often takes to heal disease.

Acceptance of a label is often the catalyst that sparks a downward spiral. It locks us in space and time, in a mental and emotional cage. As we can see from the above, a refusal to let the diagnosis dictate your belief system and desire for healing allows for unfettered life force to find its way to healing. It has been well documented that thoughts, attitudes and emotions affect our health positively as well as negatively (Braden, Lipton). Your thoughts and focus determine your behavior. If you know you are going to lose, why bother with the effort? If you feel you can win, you will invest the time and energy to do so. Winning athletes use this strategy as they mentally prepare and visualize their performance.

As a culture, we have been conditioned to expect the immediate effect of a pharmaceutical drug, and that the drug will do the healing work. There are misconceptions that the remedies or therapies will do the same work as the drug but in a "natural" way. This can be one of the shortcomings of natural medicine and quite often a roadblock. While an herb in its whole, natural form works without the side effects that often accompany the isolates in pharmacological drugs, they are still an adjunct to the healing process. Therapeutics, synthetic or natural, do not produce a cure. To effect true healing, any therapy or remedy must work with the vital force, which then enables healing.

It must provide for unrestricted flow of the energy systems in the body to regain homeostasis. Natural and energy therapies work to remove impedances to the vital force so the body can do its own healing.

Surgery, radiation and drug therapy only remove the end product of the disease process. No sane person denies that any of these may be necessary when a disease process is so far advanced that recovery may not be possible without it. If the disease process is stealing valuable energy from the host to the point that the vital force is unable to reestablish balance without these interventions, we are fortunate to have them and this is where conventional medicine shines. However, many complications arise subsequent to these treatments. Removing pathological abnormalities or administering synthetic drugs to palliate symptoms does not correct the underlying process that allowed the condition to develop initially. Removing a tumor or a cyst does not address its origin. The original cause of the imbalance must be addressed in order to shape a different, healthier outcome. This necessitates an understanding of all possible influences that may affect the vital force and lead to imbalance and ill health.

Nutrition, hydration, environment, chemical toxins, heavy metals, emotions, or philosophical beliefs – any of these can present an obstacle to a cure. If any of these obstacles remain to drive the imbalance, this lays the groundwork for the imbalance to produce symptoms elsewhere in the body. Addressing these underlying issues is the domain of a natural health practitioner illustrating why healing must be a collaborative effort between conventional and natural medicine.

A few clinical cases will further illustrate these concepts.

Lauren made an appointment to address digestive

complaints. Supplements and remedies began correcting her internal environment, helping to alleviate some of her physical symptoms. This was essential, as it can be incredibly difficult to address deeper core issues without a strong physical foundation. Time was also spent correcting her dietary indiscretions. When the body is filled with toxic chemicals from what sometimes passes as food, hormones and neurotransmitters no longer function optimally, making it difficult to think clearly and make life-supporting decisions. Initial intervention with nutrition and supplements helped, but Lauren's progress was slow. She had seen numerous doctors and had taken it upon herself to try a few interventions based on the advice of the "television gurus". Nothing, she claimed, made a real difference for very long. She arrived for one appointment at the beginning of May.

"This time of year is always the worst. Springtime...everyone starts wearing lighter clothes...it's harder to hide the weight." I could see her struggling, trying to lift the lid on something she wasn't sure she wanted to uncover. "And then there is Mother's Day," she sneered.

"No fond memories?" I inquired.

She looked at me in exasperation. " I hated my mother".

"Hate is a pretty strong word," I commented.

"Well you didn't know my mother. If you did you would probably hate her too."

"Why?"

"Because mothers are supposed to protect their children, but she couldn't even protect herself. Too busy taking care of him."

"Who? Your father?" I asked.

"Makes me sick to even call him that. I was glad when he died. I was finally free."

Ok, I thought, now the real work starts; the real healing can begin.

"Stay in touch with that anger," I told her. "That is the key to your freedom. Once we free that energy that has been smoldering there all these years, you are going to soar."

"Hold on to it? Everyone else tells me I have to let to go and forgive!"

"You're not ready to let it go. You haven't found the gift locked inside." I said.

She stared at me incredulously, "You're the craziest doctor I've ever seen." So, I asked her to follow this Mad Hatter down the rabbit hole on a journey of healing, and a chance to rewrite the story of her life. Lauren's father, a prominent political figure, had sexually abused her from an early age. Her mother chose to deny Lauren's allegations, as these would have threatened the social position of the family. She buried the anger and shame deep within believing it was neatly locked away.

Since some of her physical discomfort had been alleviated with herbal and natural remedies, she then felt empowered to deal with the underlying issue that continued to wreak havoc on her vital force. In fact, she asked, "Do you think all of the anger I was unable to voice as a child is contributing to this illness?" Such intuitive brilliance - when we seek hard enough, we will find the answers within ourselves. If there is a will, there is a way. By choosing to hold onto the anger, she felt vindicated - for if she gave it up, she would become weak and he would win. It became a reason to put up walls, to remain buried inside, to avoid feeling the pain that was paradoxically the pathway to release and growth. She began to realize this raging fire was burning everything in its path and the strategy was no longer working. With tremendous courage, she surrendered to the process.

Homeopathic remedies helped to release the shock and the energy of righteous indignation from the violation she had suffered. This shifted her perspective. A plan was developed with physical exercises that allowed for an appropriate release of anger. At her next visit, she appeared different physically, softer and a bit more settled. Lauren said she just "felt different…better."

Previously, her energy system presented with inflammation and impedance in the Liver and Gallbladder meridians. The Liver meridian processes anger and the Gallbladder resentment. Laurel's seething anger kept fueling the fire of inflammation in her digestive system, resulting in a myriad of problems. In a few short weeks, the energy impedance and inflammation in her Liver and Gallbladder meridians were restored to a more balanced level. She now declares, "I can honestly say this is the best I've felt my whole life." Lauren's attitude has changed from resignation and depression to gratitude and a renewed vigor for life. She is pleased that she "stumbled" on natural medicine, and states that is she is grateful for the way it has profoundly changed her life.

Because a particular set of remedies worked for Laurel does not mean it can be applied across the board to clients with similar complaints. This is the difficulty in implementing natural medicine into our current Western framework for treatments. The conventional system scarcely allows for individualized analysis and treatment. Rather, we are grouped and streamlined into a one-fits-most scenario in the interest of time and profitability.

And in another case: Mary arrived at my office with digestive issues and a medical diagnosis similar to Lauren's. However, initial testing revealed a radically different energetic signature than Lauren. Both had been prescribed similar drugs through the years, yet neither experienced anything other than temporary relief. The major energy disruptions for Mary were sourced in the Spleen/Stomach meridians and her Triple Warmer (endocrine system).

Two years prior to the development of symptoms Mary experienced a particularly stressful time. She had lost her job, was having difficulty in her marriage and her father, with whom she was very close, died suddenly. Mary informed me that severe anxiety during her childhood would bring on diarrhea. The episodes of diarrhea began shortly after her grandmother, who watched her after school, died. A neighbor was then assigned to after-school care. The situation was extremely stressful as the neighbor was dictatorial and frightened her. She could not speak her mind and buried her anger; she felt trapped and unable to escape. She was planning to leave her husband and move home with her father, but lost both her job and her father in the same year. Again, she experienced feeling trapped and unable to escape.

Medical intervention would temporarily alleviate her symptoms, however, the cause of her illness was still running in the background and eventually, the symptoms would return. Clearly, she told me, her current therapy was not addressing her disease so she was seeking another path to heal.

Addressing the underlying cause of illness in both of these cases required tackling the energetic imprint and dysfunctional thought patterns programmed in the body. The recent events in Mary's life mimicked an earlier traumatic experience, "booting up" old programming that allowed her to survive at the time. As a child, rather than lash out at her caregiver and incite further wrath, she buried her rage to prevent her life being threatened. But she lacked the ability to concentrate in school, as she constantly worried about everything. She also admitted being angry with her parents for placing her in a threatening situation. The pattern of shutting down and avoidance that worked for her as a child was no longer working for her as an adult. She felt helpless to change the pattern as it evoked such a deep, visceral response. The traumatic situations of her childhood had upset the balance of her vital force, and this energy remained stored in her mind as well as her body. The strategy that allowed her to survive as a child was no longer working in her adult life.

Taking remedies that were homeopathic to her symptoms changed Mary's perspective from feeling trapped to knowing that she could now make different choices. Instead of feeling stuck and ruminating over everything, the blocked energy in her Stomach (and Spleen/Pancreas) was freed, allowing Mary's body to utilize it to heal.

From these stories, we see two critical points depicting the necessity of natural medicine. First, the diagnosis of the disease only tells us of the effects. It classifies the physical manifestations of the process but gives no clue as to its origin. If only palliation of symptoms is desired, then we could rest at this point. Without addressing the origins, the actual disease process (imbalance of the vital force) continues to run in the background and true healing is highly unlikely to occur.

Evidence of the disease process was presented in the symptomatology, on mental and emotional as well as physical levels. In this, Mary and Lauren each presented very different pictures. While a few of the physical symptoms were similar, the triggers and modalities were very different. Lauren abused alcohol and became verbally abusive; Mary was so consumed with worry, she became overwhelmed and unable to complete the tasks of daily life. Mary felt better after eating; Lauren was worse. While Mary was fearful of being alone, Lauren needed time to herself. Lauren was always too warm, even in the winter; Mary was always chilly, even in the summer.

Perhaps the greatest difference were the ghosts of the past trauma that continued to haunt both women's daily existence. Appearing to be buried in the past and long forgotten, nothing could be further from the truth. Early images and imprints continued to walk with them, coloring their every decision and waking hours. To expand on our "programming" metaphor, these experiences were continuing to run in the background, greatly hindering achievement of their goals and dreams. It was extremely difficult for either woman to enjoy life fully in the present moment. Unresolved shocks and traumas produce problems over time, and very often are an integral part of chronic diseases.

CHAPTER 7

THE ELEMENTS OF THE WHEEL

"Have you noticed that in the forest nothing grows in a straight line?" asks the old sage. "Curves and whorls dominate the natural course of growth, patterns are cyclical and repeat." Together they watch the clouds drift over the lake that sits behind the ancient medicine wheel. Though simple in its format, the energy from the wheel is palpable, and humbling, whispering its sacred nature deep directly into Bendith. As the wind shifted so did the emotions of the healer. As if the sage can see right into the healer's soul he says, *"It is the mind that creates the suffering. It is the mind that creates the illusion of separation.*

"All emotion," quips the sage , *"are the very essence of humanity, what makes us uniquely human. E-motions, are simply energy in motion. They are what unite*

and separate, cause growth or decay, create illness and healing. It is wise to remember that this energy remains in motion; it is the mind patterns that stagnate causing suffering. Within each of your painful experiences lies your greatest path to power"

The old sage points to Arwyn standing at the edge of a pristine lake, calm, reflective. Glancing over, she acknowledges our presence to come forward, the smell of sweet grass and sage rising from the shell in her hand. Motioning toward the water, arms and face lifted to the sun, the old sage explains that Arwyn is making prayers, her connection through earth to the Source of All Potential, to Great Mystery, the Tao. Not reciting obligatory words from memory designed to dispel fear, doubt and worry. Making prayers. Lifting energy, the life force from the earth pulling it through her body, melding it with the cells of her body, adding individualized expressions of life force. She breathes deeply, then releases with gentleness onto the wind, combined with the resonance of song to create a new frequency. Life force drawn through nature, altered by desire, by will, and released in altered frequency back to nature. And through her song, transfers frequencies from her heart, harmonic patterns that resonate with and magnify the electromagnetic patterns of nature.

"To make prayers from a position of fear or worry," she says, " dampens the energy; it makes the energy heavy and releases chaotic and stagnant patterns into the ethers. To make prayers, we create our realities - harmonic or chaotic - based on how we use these energies of nature."

"To know the light you must understand the dark; to know the dark you must understand the light. We live in a dual universe that encompasses polar opposites. Yet each pole contains within itself the opposite and a path of neutrality. When exactly does it cease to be day and become night?"

The sage stops at the East Gate. "The Wheel is circular, without beginning or end; no one place more exalted than another. All is interwoven and interdependent on optimal energy flow through each section." The old sage emphasizes again that man is part of nature, neither above nor below; rather inextricably linked. Nature holds everything in balance; an innate wisdom flows though striving for harmony.

This system is rooted in a premise of wholeness. Balance is a natural state; illness is simply a deviation from this harmony. Suffering and strife are rooted in this alienation from the whole. The ancient philosophy of the five paths is based on observation of nature. The framework assists the healer to determine where the natural flow of energy has been disrupted, inhibiting the innate wisdom for healing.

After pause for reflection, and burning of the sacred herbs for purification, the sage leads Bendith to the Wheel. "Here we turn inward, drawing down into the depths of the silence to a place we will call still point, the pause between the inbreath and the outbreath, that point of silent suspension, the origin of infinite possibility." The old sage unravels the flow by explaining how commencing at birth, nature waits in anticipation for the infant to draw its first breath, the breath that first enters the body at the dawn of its life and is the last to leave at the end. The Ancients say that in that breath we draw the energy that animates the clay. Yet even prior to that, the vital force moves upon the waters of the womb, igniting the will – the will to be, the will to thrive. Thus begin the teachings, older than written history, yet as fundamental to healing insight now at the dawn of time.

THE WHEEL OF THE FIVE ELEMENTS

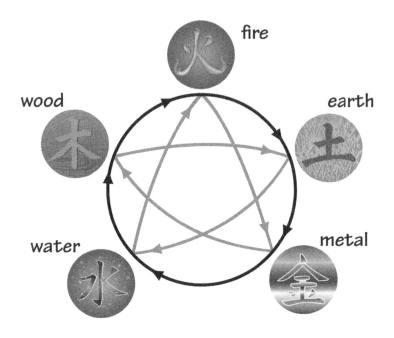

In the following section, as in convention, the names of the meridians are in all capital, to differentiate from the organ (i.e. KIDNEY for the meridian, and Kidney for the organ)

WATER

Season	Winter
Meridian	*KIDNEY / BLADDER*
Emotion	*Fear*
Gift	*Willpower, Courage and Instinct*
Spiritual Element	*Wisdom*

WATER - Where our inspiration fires our Will, our will to be, to do, and to thrive. Ancient alchemists tell us that Water is the root of all matter. Life begins in the waters of the womb. We are born from water, are composed of mostly water and water is critical for life. Water nourishes and is the home of our Will Power – that which provides us with the capacity to express our unique gifts and talents, to achieve our goals and desires. We use our will to feed the creative desires and to shape our life path through the material world around us.

Fear is the adversary of our Will, with the potential to freeze forward movement. Water extinguishes Fire, dampening, even drowning our courage and passion. Fear, anxiety, apprehension, dread – all thwart the progress, turning the energy inside. Retreating versus doing deprives the world of your unique abilities. Know that even in the depths of winter, when all growth appears to cease, movement is occurring deep within the earth. When frozen, daydreaming restores warmth, melting immobilization, as does gratitude for our many blessings. If nothing else, have gratitude for your breath that gives life.

KIDNEY is the seat of the Life-essence, the pilot light of the body. The highest expression of a balanced KIDNEY is Wisdom. KIDNEY processes beginnings and endings, birth and death, and is the carrier of our genetic make-up. KIDNEY also rules formation of bones and teeth, and encompasses the kidneys and bladder.

WOOD

Season	*Spring*
Meridian	*LIVER / GALLBLADDER*
Emotion	*Anger*
Gift	Vision, Direction, Reason, Courage
Spiritual Element	*Benevolence, Discernment*

WOOD - The energy is the rapid pulse of spring surging forth. The forces that had been stored in the roots and seeds burst forth with prolific vigor. The world is in a state of rapid transformation. Here we have the creative vision, the planning and revising that reinvents the physical world around us. A clear vision of our path feeds the Fire of our courage and passions to move forward and make changes.

Wood feeds the desire to express our unique essence with enthusiasm.

Discipline needs cultivation here as bursting forth without balance can deplete our vitality. Pushing blindly forward without the balance of mental discipline can upset the stability and security of our projects. We use discretion to dole out the proper amounts of energy at the right time. Lack of planning and vision upsets stability and natural rhythm, leading to frustration, anger and resentment - as well as rash decisions. Wood out of control can destroy what we have established as solid, stable and working. This includes our emotional as well as our physical environment. When the outward expression of creative enthusiasm is thwarted or suppressed, this energy turns inward, resulting in various forms of depression. Taking the time to assess direction, gaining clarity and a vision for your life's purpose (Wood) will feed the Fire of the heart to create a life that is positively affirming with forward momentum. Meditation stills the mind, returning an internal locus of control and with it, imagination and positive direction.

The highest expression of LIVER is solid self-worth, vision and purposeful direction to achieve goals and missions in a benevolent manner. Physically, the liver filters and stores blood and chi, the gallbladder stores bile, and both are associated with the health of the blood, muscle, tendons, and nails.

FIRE

Season	Summer
Meridian	HEART / SMALL INTESTINE PERICARDIUM / TRIPLE WARMER
Emotion	*Joy*
Gift	*Love, Insight, Inspiration, Vitality*
Spiritual Element	*Compassion*

FIRE – The passion and inspiration to create change in our world. Inspiration and desires in alignment with the will to facilitate the flow of life through the energy grid of the body. HEART stores the Spirit, and allows our ability for connection and compassion with all of life. It nourishes the blood and shines the light of love on our perceptions. When balanced, we operate with appropriate behavior, timely interactions, and connect in dialogue. HEART fires the rhythm and flow of energy, the balance of natural oscillations of life in alignment with nature. Our heart energy affects those within our sphere of influence.

When the HEART is disturbed, the symptoms include forgetfulness, lack of connection with others, and an absence of joy. When shock upsets the rhythm, stagnation sets in and results in the halting of vibrations, which is inimical to life. Imbalances can cause insomnia, anxiety and hypertension.

SMALL INTESTINE, the partner of HEART, separates the pure from the impure physically, as well as emotionally and spiritually. It is associated with the ability to separate thoughts and beliefs, truths and, confidence to in one's own judgment.

Physically the HEART includes the heart, blood and vessels and the thymus gland; the SMALL INTESTINE includes the small intestines. The highest of HEART expression is a universal love, compassion and connection with all of life.

PERICARDIUM sets the pace, the rhythm, and protects the heart from insults and attacks.

This center fires the TRIPLE WARMER as the energy through the meridians stimulates the endocrine organs to release life-affirming hormones. TRIPLE WARMER establishes, maintains and regulates the flow through endocrine organs. Change in energy will affect the hormonal output of the gland. This then communicates chemically to the organs, tissues and cells. When will, mind and heart are aligned, creation occurs as we move foreword and receive feedback for growth and evolution.

Physically, the PERICARDIUM does not have an anatomical component and is often misunderstood. TRIPLE WARMER encompasses the endocrine organs. The highest expression of a balanced PERICARDIUM /

TRIPLE WARMER is balance and rhythm that supports vitality and love of living.

METAL

Season	*Autumn*
Meridian	LUNG / LARGE INTESTINE
Emotion	*Grief*
Gift	Transformation, Release, Gift of Life
Spiritual Element	Appreciation, Gratitude of Present Moment

METAL –Breath, inspiration, spark of life. The vital energy utilizes minerals of the earth as a grounding source. The ability to embrace the present moment and understand the ephemeral nature of life defines a balanced LUNG meridian. It is the ground for inspiration and intuition. When inspiration is lacking, the creative drive is depleted and energy turns inward, withdrawing deeply as in autumn when the life force draws back down into the earth to prepare for winter.

Grief disrupts and even stops breath; drawing deep breath can cause physical pain. It rearranges time and priorities. Grief teaches us the ephemeral nature of life, the precious gift that is our life. In this natural but very painful turn of the wheel we experience meaning in, and respect for, all life. Mired in profound depths of grief, it is possible only to deal with what is immediately in the present. This shines light on the precious value of the present moment, reminding us that nothing is permanent or can be taken for granted. A profound sense of compassion can be cultivated as we empathize with this pain that is common to all humanity.

Change can occur in an instant. Values often radically change. We constantly reassess where and with whom we invest our time and energy. Lessons of surrender happen here. At times the pain is so great we stop breathing; to breathe hurts because the breath pulls the vital force through the body. We are challenged to release the past and the future and remain with the breath in the current moments. It is vitally important, though often avoided, to stay centered and just breathe. Feelings then are unbound and can move through the body instead of being stuck, only to wreak havoc later.

Take walks in the woods or along the water's edge; let the healing power of Nature be a balm to the soul. Through pausing and reflection we can find our way to a place of still point, staying with centered breath. From here, decide what no longer works; eliminate or let go to create space for something to enter. Then the process begins again, with new wisdom and new experience connecting breath with the spirit of vital force to re-start the cycle.

The highest expression of a balanced LUNG / LARGE INTESTINE is the gift of the preciousness of the present moment, the source of power. LARGE INTESTINE surrenders that which is toxic and no longer serves our highest good, physically as well as figuratively. Physically LUNG includes lungs and the respiratory system; LARGE INTESTINE the large intestine and eliminatory system.

EARTH

Season	Late Summer
Meridian	SPLEEN / STOMACH
Emotion	Worry
Gift	Intention, Integrity, Manifestation
Spiritual Element	Devotion

EARTH – Where we digest and assimilate experiences, the cauldron of manifestation. When healthy, SPLEEN finds balance in consideration of options, possibilities and making decisions. When unbalanced, a lack of motivation ensues. We can become stuck in the muck of rumination halting forward movement. Excess sympathy, worry and doubt will stagnate the vital force. This tends to crystallize and impede patterns of thought, speech and action. Left unchecked, disengagement from life or creative endeavors occurs. We begin to question, doubt and worry which leads to procrastination, unfinished projects, and a feeling of defeat.

SPLEEN /STOMACH is the meridian of transformation and transportation, ruling physical and energetic nourishment. STOMACH governs digestion and absorption; it ripens and rots, procuring nourishment and separating waste. SPLEEN gathers and stores the vital energy (chi) from our food. As we digest and assimilate, the world we created is made manifest.

Devotion to our chosen purpose or mission is the highest expression of SPLEEN. Our vital force is channeled into manifesting our physical and spiritual goals and desires. The PANCREAS allows for the enjoyment of the sweetness of life and its many gifts. When following our life path and all is in alignment, this positively feeds and then affects the immune system via the SPLEEN. Physically, SPLEEN encompasses the spleen and pancreas; STOMACH encompasses the stomach and esophagus.

CHAPTER 8

THE HEALING POWER OF MAN'S ENERGY

"If you want to find the secrets of the universe, think in terms of energy, frequency and vibration." Nikola Tesla

And, if you want to uncover the secrets of healing, seek to understand the energy systems of man. Ultimately, we are energy manifesting as matter. The energy body is primary, the material body secondary as a manifestation of energy. And, here is perhaps one of the best-kept secrets in medicine: *the bioenergy of the human body can be accessed and studied objectively.* Changing states of the energy body can be detected, observed, and measured. Although in the early stages of scientifically understanding the complexities and intricacies of the energy body, we can witness its effects on the material realm.

After developing bladder cancer in the 1940's, German medical doctor Reinhold Voll sought alternative answers for his own healing through Traditional Chinese Medicine. Success in reversing this illness changed the trajectory of his work. Voll spent twenty years researching the meridian system, and discovered that electrically conductive points on the skin corresponded with specific internal organs of the body. Further research lead to the discovery of a connection between the electrical conductance and the physiological state of the organs associated with that meridian. With the assistance of Fritz Werner, an electrical engineer, Dr. Voll devised a system to study these acupuncture pathways. A method was devised that combined the fundamentals of acupuncture with modern electronics. Originally called Electro Acupuncture according to Voll (EAV), it is now more commonly known as Electro Dermal Analysis (or EDA) to reflect its ability to provide an analysis.

Extensive research by several practitioners proved the value of this form of testing for pre-diagnostic screening. EAV testing provides the ability to record progress over time, providing objective proof of the efficacy of therapy – whether conventional or energetic. Perhaps most importantly, Dr. Voll did not recommend this testing to replace traditional methods of diagnosis and therapy; rather he advocated for this to compliment conventional, clinical work. He felt strongly that the practice of EAV should be accompanied by knowledge of anatomy and clinical medicine, as well as pharmacology (allopathic and homeopathic) and Chinese acupuncture.

It is energy that is being accessed and influenced as it flows along the acupuncture meridian network. These meridian channels are networks of energetic flow and communication, connecting organ systems throughout the body. Meridians represent the body's Internet, integrating various forms of input into a unifying whole. "Clicking" on a specific site (acupuncture point) allows access to an entire web of information. This represents an entire realm of information currently not being utilized by conventional therapies.

The practice of Electro Dermal Analysis has been the subject of controversy regarding its accuracy or relevance to the analysis of conditions based on conventional diagnosis. These concerns are unwarranted; it has been clinically proven to produce consistent, reproducible results. As regards to relevancy of medical conditions, numerous studies have been conducted that do show strong correlations with standard conventional analysis, including a landmark study published in 2003, which demonstrated a 99% correlation between the EAV - measured abnormalities and patients with Chronic Inflammatory Demyelinating Polyneuropathy disease (Ericcson, Pittaway, & Lai). Additional research by Drs. Tsuei and Lam, Voll, and Madill revealed correlations in EDA testing and diabetes mellitus, as well as inflammation, gastrointestinal issues and chronic degenerative diseases. The article, *Bio-Energetic Medicine: The Past, Present and Future of the ElectroDermal Screening System,* states that Dr. Tsuei and colleagues completed over twenty studies using EAV. In the first study she states: "Conditions seen included peptic ulcers, appendicitis, chronic chorea, and cancer of the colon, breast and uterus. In every case, readings taken with EAV matched standard diagnostic tests." Dr. Tsuei provided a theoretical basis for EAV. All living creatures generate energy containing biological information, giving rise to a resonance with a direct relationship between quality of organ function and the energy generated.

Archeological records indicate knowledge of acupuncture meridians as far back as 1600 BC. Several texts such as *Nei Ching* (2600 BC), the *Canon of Medicine* (475 BC) and the *Analytical Dictionary of Characters* (206 BC) describe the meridian channels, treatments, counter-indications and pathological issues. The vital energy, or chi, is distributed via the meridian networks. This chi combines with the breath and circulates through all the systems of the body in pathways called meridians, and these meridians work in conjunction with each other to control bodily processes.

The acupuncture meridians comprise an organizing network for distribution and utilization of information necessary for maintaining homeostasis. Research using SQUID (Super Quantum Interface Device) provided a means for verification of acupuncture channels. Analogous to the body's Internet, these meridians provide a system of instantaneous communication to all the various components of the body. Free flow of energy through the meridians is essential to vibrant health. Impedance in that meridian indicates distortion of coherent communication that can manifest as a physical, emotional or mental disturbance. The ability to communicate instantaneously, both locally and globally, implies coherence in the meridian network. Each meridian has its own direction of flow, and the intensity of that flow can be measured by electro diagnosis.

Since inflammatory processes begin with increased energy production, this will register as an elevation in conductance through the meridian. This inflammatory process results in an increase in the concentration of ions, which correspond to the elevation in electrical conductance. Likewise, a decrease in electrical conductance indicates an impedance of energy that could possibly lead to a degenerative condition. Energy impedance can result in an accumulation of free radicals and a decrease in oxygen levels, leading to a change in chemistry and eventually, changes in cellular manifestation.

It is important to note that EAV is not *directly* measuring the energy in the meridians of the body. Since this type of energy lies outside of the four primary forces of classical physics, direct measurement is not possible. However, when you run electricity through the acupuncture point, a bio-physiological phenomenon occurs. The electrical flow (conductance) provides an indication of the energetic health status of that specific meridian.

Readings of test subjects will provide essentially the same results for different well-trained, experienced practitioners. This establishes EAV as a valid health screening modality because the test readings are reproducible. The *American Journal of Acupuncture* has published articles regarding its valid, scientific basis for a "true and legitimate preventative medicine". The same journal published additional articles regarding the advantages in utilizing EAV: as a testing method to assist in hypoglycemia, stress and psychosomatic illness (Madill, 1980), to pre-test the efficacy of various medicines for different diseases (Voll, 1980), and to demonstrate the effectiveness for determining the correct dosage of allopathic or homeopathic medicines to treat diabetes mellitus, (Tsuei, & Zhao, 1990). Recently a practitioner in Africa, Nadejda Grigorova, published her extensive work of 11 years exploring EAV, homeopathy, quantum physics and the role of underlying viral, bacterial and fungal pathogens in diseases.

EAV empowers both the practitioner and the client by providing a system to locate the obstacles to healing within the subtle energy fields. In *Vibrational Medicine*, Gerber emphasizes the importance of this testing. The following is a summary of his work: The ability to measure electromagnetic disturbances in the meridian system and find imbalances in the flow of chi allows one to detect ongoing cellular pathology in a particular area of the body as well as predict future organic dysfunction. Electroacupuncture technologies may allow us to actually measure subtle energy imbalances that are precursors to illness. In addition, these same technologies can reveal illness in the physical body, which is still too subtle to be measured by conventional laboratory tests (Gerber, 1998).

EAV has enormous value as a predictive tool in preventative medicine. EAV has the capacity to reveal the state of energy flow and level of impedance within organ systems. It provides information as to the extent that toxins are affecting the functionality of tissues and organs. Additionally, the testing process can be utilized to determine the compatibility of remedies. Since remedies can be suited to individual needs, this increases the success of any treatment program. Also, EAV provides a screening tool to assess information regarding chemical sensitivities, environmental irritants and allergens. And finally, clients can see progress over time by witnessing the change in measurements. This serves as positive reinforcement to continue therapy.

Each meridian has it own "anatomy", so when energy is disrupted or impeded in that channel, changes will manifest in the electrical fields. Through testing, we can detect, measure and monitor this disruption of energy. When the disruption or impedance persists, the body will reflect that disruption through manifesting a change in mental, emotional or physical ways.

This mirrors what Hahnemann stated in his work *The Organon of Medicine*: when the vital force is disrupted, a disturbance becomes evident by observing the effects on the organism. These effects or symptoms (on mental, emotional, physical or spiritual levels) are viewed as the disease. Yet, as we see here, there is a change that precedes these symptoms, a change in the dynamic realm. From the perspective of natural medicine, we are interested in the changes that occurred, the changes that impinged upon the vital force, which then result in the derangement. This cause of the derangement is what is to be addressed as the disease in process. Symptoms can be quelled, but this practice does not necessarily re-establish homeostasis that leads to vibrant health. Instead, a type of equilibrium around a dysfunction results that allows us to continue functioning while the programming error still runs in the background. The energy dysfunction remains.

Changes occur primarily in the energy system, then manifest in the material body as physical or chemical changes. Energy manifesting through chemistry is energy "in formation", a change in energy leads to a change in chemistry. A change in chemistry leads to a change in form. This is simple to comprehend when we observe this phenomena occurring in nature.

During winter, flower bulbs lay dormant waiting for the return of spring. As winter's blanket slowly melts, plants deep in the earth begin to stir from slumber. Gradual changes in energy drift seamlessly from one season into the next. These shifting of energies are a harbinger for changing seasons. Daylight lengthens, temperature builds slowly, winds shift, and all these changes in energy provide information to the seed. The change in energy informs the seed that it is time to switch the program from dormancy to activity. The shift in energy warms the Earth around the bulb, preparing an environment conducive for growth, and precipitates changes in chemistry to initiate new growth. There is a change in energy prior to the manifestation of any physical changes.

We recognize the approach of a storm by sensing environmental change in temperature, humidity, and wind. These changes in energy provide information that a shift is coming. Our bodies recognize similar, numerous energy shifts occurring every moment in our external and internal environments. In addition to our five senses, each cell is an organ of perception wired to perceive even the slightest change. The cell "analyzes" these shifts in the environment and responds accordingly.

These shifts cause energy changes either locally or globally through the connective tissue matrix system of the body. Scientific studies confirm that this initial change occurs faster than the speed of electrical nerve transmission. Evidence points to these changes in energy being communicated at light speed along the meridian networks that run through the connective tissue system. The energy changes are then registered as electrical changes in the nervous system, which in turn signal chemical (enzymatic) changes that affect chemical and physical changes.

The energy flow through the meridians provides a wealth of information to the practitioner of natural medicine as to the health of the body. When flow through the meridians is interrupted, it disrupts our internal balance, hampering our defenses or ability to adapt to a wide variety of situations. When healthy, the body as a whole and every cell possess a variety of possible responses and adaptations to the change. Ultimately, the change in energy (the change in information) expresses physically in the form of a material change.

In his second book on subtle energies, *Life Force, the Scientific Basis*, Claude Swanson describes the meridian network as a communication system, linking all cells and organs in all parts of the body. Research has uncovered that the meridian system also transports DNA, RNA and mitochondrial material, which may provide undifferentiated stem cells to help with tissue repair (Swanson, 2010, p. 140). Swanson provides a summary of the work conducted by Korean scientist Kim Bonghan in the 1960s proving the existence of a duct system that follows the meridian channels. Also known as the Bonghan ducts, their existence was verified by injecting a radioactive tracer into the ducts and following it through the acupuncture system. These ducts were filled with a fluid which when analyzed were found to contain high quantities of DNA and RNA. The experiments of Dr. Kwang-Sup Soh in 2004 propose a model for how the bioenergy flows through the meridian network. Dr. Soh proposes that the DNA in the meridian channels absorb and re-emit biophotons (quantum packets of energy) which travel the network and act as boosting signals. This proposal is supported by the revolutionary research of Dr. Fritz Popp whose work demonstrates that biophotons play a key role in the regulation, development and differentiation of cells. Moreover, the biophoton field (i.e. energy, quantum energy) precedes and directs chemical and physical processes.

The following section contains a summary of the twelve acupuncture meridians, their partners and associations as well as the manifestations that result from balance and imbalance. Entire books have been written on this subject so this provides only a brief summary, to introduce the breadth and depth of information that is available. For more complete information, consult *The Web That Has No Weaver: Understanding Chinese Medicine*, by Ted Kaptchuk, or *Between Heaven and Earth: A Guide to Chinese Medicine,* by Beinfield and Korngold. Again, as in convention, capital letters denote the meridian system, i.e. KIDNEY, to differentiate from the organ, i.e. kidney.

The Twelve Acupuncture Meridians

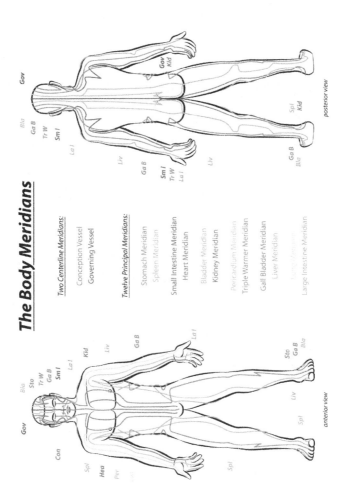

LIVER

The physical function of the LIVER meridian is to filter and store blood and chi, and is responsible for the health of the blood, muscle, tendons, and nails. Physical issues associated with an imbalanced Liver are disorders of the liver and gallbladder, pain, swelling breast, lumps, stiff joints or tendons, muscle spasms, poor memory, dizziness, splitting headaches, red face & eyes, dry mouth, tinnitus. LIVER governs blood, menses, blood sugar and pressure imbalances, and autoimmune disorders. A balanced LIVER meridian leads to a healthy sense of self-worth, acceptance and adaptability to change. In an unbalanced state LIVER is associated with anger, frustration, unhealthy boundaries, emotional tension and stress, spasmodic movement, aggression and an inability to control rage.

GALLBLADDER

The GALLBLADDER meridian is the Yang aspect of the element of Wood, and also Spring. A balanced GALLBLADDER is the ground for "Courage & Decision"; it carries out the orders of the General (LIVER). An imbalance leads to timidity and fear of places and things, as well as anger and rash decisions. The Gallbladder is the largest meridian in the body, covering a number of organs and areas. Physical issues associated are those that pertain to the liver and gallbladder, bile and ducts, as well as disorders that occur along this meridian: ear (tinnitus, deafness), eye (glaucoma, night blindness), head (vertigo & migraines), neck, chest, and joints.

LUNG

To understand the ephemeral nature of life defines a balanced LUNG meridian. It is the ground for inspiration and intuition. Unresolved grief and the inability to see the delicate, temporal nature of life can create an imbalance in the LUNG. Other symptoms of imbalance include feelings of restlessness, erratic behavior, dissatisfaction, an incompletion in life and being easily annoyed. Respiratory disorders, asthma and breathing difficulties are associated with LUNG imbalance along with skin, vascular, neck, nose, erratic behavior, and cough. LUNG is associated with the sense of smell and instinctive judgments.

LARGE INTESTINE

This meridian "Moves the Turbid" and rules elimination, and is connected with the thyroid. On a physical level it absorbs water and trace minerals from the body's waste. An inability to let go on any level - physically, mentally, emotionally or spiritually - can lead to an imbalance of this meridian. Symptoms of imbalance include constipation or diarrhea, abdominal pain, as well as frozen shoulder, trigeminal neuralgia or facial paralysis, and thyroid disorders.

SPLEEN (PANCREAS)

The spleen and pancreas are considered jointly in this meridian. SPLEEN is the meridian of "Transformation & Transportation" and rules digestion and absorption. It moves energy upward to LUNGS, mouth & lips. When healthy, SPLEEN finds a balance in consideration of options, possibilities and making decisions. When unbalanced, a lack of motivation and excitement, disengagement in either life or creativity ensues. This also creates stagnation, defeatism, excessive worry, procrastination, unfinished projects, and a feeling of being trapped. Diseases that can occur along this path include gastrointestinal distention, pain, bloating, diarrhea, sugar metabolism and appetite disorders. Chronic bleeding disorders and hemorrhoids can also ensue.

STOMACH

The STOMACH "Receives and Ripens", sending the pure to the SPLEEN. An imbalance in STOMACH may include disorders of the stomach and abdominal organs. When the descending function is impaired and directing energy upwards – nausea, stomachache, distention, belching, vomiting, even chest discomfort can occur.

HEART

The HEART "Stores the Spirit", and allows our ability for connection and compassion with all of life. It nourishes the blood and shines the light of love on our perceptions. When balanced, we operate with appropriate behavior, timely interactions, and connect in dialogue. When the HEART is disturbed, the symptoms include forgetfulness, lack of connection with others, and an absence of joy. Long-standing imbalances can produce agitation, aggression and hostility. Physical imbalances include disorders of the heart, blood and vessels, tachycardia, arrhythmia, anemia and hypertension. Other possible disturbances include stuttering, tremors and psychosomatic disorders, anxiety disorders, insomnia, fatigue, dizziness, situational anxiety and mental illness.

SMALL INTESTINE

SMALL INTESTINE is the meridian that "Separates Pure from Impure". It is associated with the ability to separate thoughts and beliefs, truths and trusting in one's own judgment. SMALL INTESTINE transmits the pure essences to the SPLEEN and sends the remainder for elimination to the BLADDER AND LARGE INTESTINE. Disorders along this pathway include abdominal pain, intestinal rumblings, irritable bowel syndrome, diarrhea, constipation, stiffness of neck and cervical spondylitis.

PERICARDIUM (CIRCULATION)

The "Heart Protector" protects the heart from over-stimulation and shock. It is also associated with the screening of psychic impulses. A balanced PERICARDIUM generates a smooth, rhythmic pulse and blood pressure. Imbalances in this meridian include anxiety, heart palpitations, upper abdominal issues, morning sickness ulcers and mental disorders. An imbalance may also manifest as being impulsive, the inability to follow through on commitments, and vacillating between being too trusting and the inability to trust.

TRIPLE WARMER (TRIPLE HEATER)

The Endocrine system is represented through the TRIPLE WARMER. It directs the relationship between organs that regulate water, mediating between Water and Fire. It distributes chi and regulates the organs and the hormones. TRIPLE WARMER, as its name implies, divides into three sections: Upper includes everything from the lungs upward and regulates blood circulation, respiration and water in the lungs; the Middle includes everything between the diaphragm and the navel - spleen, pancreas, stomach and gallbladder; and the Lower from the naval down – liver, large and small intestine, kidney, bladder and reproductive organs. In addition to hormonal disorders, others include: ear disorders; pain, paralysis and polyneuropathy of upper extremity, frozen shoulder and pain in back of chest, constipation, disorders of the eye and of the temporal region.

KIDNEY

KIDNEY "Stores the Will"; it is the seat of the Life-essence, the pilot light of the body and the root of Water (Yin) and Fire (Yang). A balanced KIDNEY is the "Seat of Wisdom", and the ability to process the cycles of birth, maturation and death; beginnings and endings. KIDNEY also carries inherited characteristics and governs development both physically and sexually. Impedance in this meridian can lead to either Yin or Yang deficiencies. Imbalance in KIDNEY can produce existential anxiety, dread of death, and inability to age gracefully, as well as lack of being assertive, being controlled easily by others, taking blame and feeling guilt. Physical disturbances include: reproductive and developmental disorders such as impotence, sterility, genito-urinary system, birth defects, and mental retardation. KIDNEY rules the formation of bones and teeth. Physical issues also include tinnitus, convulsions, fainting, dizziness, alopecia, ear disorders, and bronchial asthma.

BLADDER

This meridian receives and excretes urine, and stores and eliminates waste. BLADDER receives chi from KIDNEY, which it uses to transform and eliminate fluids. Imbalances in the meridian include disorders along the bladder pathway. Since this travels up the back of the body, back and neck pain are often associated with impedance in this meridian. Other issues include bladder and genital disorders, incontinence, burning urination, muscle cramps and excessive phlegm.

CHAPTER 9

A QUANTUM BLUEPRINT FOR HEALING

In the 1920's, an event occurred that was never supposed to happen. The infamous Double Slit experiment revealed that particles of matter were not static; rather "matter" could behave as either a particle or a wave, depending upon how it was being observed. Our stable, solid world gave way to an underlying sea of quantum energy fields. The simplest known particles of matter possessed characteristics of solid particles and of fluid waves. Scientists, unable to reconcile this behavior within the accepted laws of Newtonian physics, adopted a new theory called *wave-particle duality*. This remained a hotbed of debate within the field of physics as a framework was sought to understand this inexplicable behavior. Since no logical explanation could be concluded at that time, this finding became an accepted paradox within the realm of physics.

Thus began a radically new way of attempting to

understand the world, with the birth of Quantum Mechanics. It seemed that a whole new set of principles apart from classical physics were operating at the subatomic level. This realm operated beyond the four fundamental forces of classical physics, which are electromagnetic, gravitational, strong and weak nuclear forces. Researcher William Tiller, spoke of these "subtle energies" as existing beyond the four classical known forces. This information compels a transformation in conventional understanding of the whole of man to accommodate the subtle energy body.

The idea that subtle energy can be quantified strictly in electromagnetic terms would be an erroneous supposition. While the human body does generate electromagnetic fields that can be observed, it would be incorrect to assume the energy systems of the meridians are also electromagnetic. The Super Quantum Interface Device (SQUID) has proved otherwise, demonstrating communication within meridians to be nonlocal and discontinuous – and faster than the speed of light. To postulate that the infinitesimal amount of data that we receive at every moment is received, directed and communicated strictly through electromagnetic and chemical means is no longer logical, nor rational. However, these subtle energies have yet to be apprehended or directly measured due to the limits of our current technology, which is also based on the four known forces. And, although at one point X-rays and gamma rays could not be measured, their effects on matter could be observed. We find ourselves at this very crossroad when exploring the subtle energy systems of man. We do not have the means to directly measure them, yet we can observe their effects on the physical realm.

Energy fields have been an integral part of healing since antiquity, only recently being eclipsed by the development of cell theory, microbiology and pharmacology. The mechanical/chemical model has served to advance our study and knowledge of medicine, yet it is simply one explanation. Our error resides in the acceptance of its corollary, which is "this currently sanctioned system to the exclusion of all others". If healing is the ultimate objective of a healthcare system, can we afford to ignore or turn our backs on the rich information available in the subtle energy body? Man is multidimensional and we need to view health care from a different, more holistic perspective. We have physical specialists, mental and emotional specialists, so why not energetic specialists to assess the health of the vital energy body? If we continue to attempt manipulating health from a purely material perspective, we will miss key information that can positively direct the healing process. It is time to reintroduce and integrate the traditional healing methods of energy medicine with our current practice. If these methods were ineffective, then cultures without conventional medicine would have perished many millennia ago.

In his book *Life Force; the Scientific Basis*, Claude Swanson details the extensive scientific research in subtle energy and energy medicine occurring around the world. Swanson states that this energy that is currently being overlooked by conventional physics constitutes a "fifth force". He concludes that this Life Force is like no other force known to science responds to consciousness and alters the other basic laws of physics. The life force is involved with processes pivotal to growth and healing, and is central to the healing arts in many cultures. Swanson asserts that this force constitutes a building energy, reversing entropy and bringing order out of chaos. Forming a bridge between the old paradigms and a new dimension of reality, this path has the potential to unify science with spirituality. An additional point that is paramount to this point of view: it has been demonstrated that the fifth force does not weaken with distance and penetrates most materials and shielding.

Russian physicist Dr. Yury Kronn teaches that only 4% of the universe is occupied by both matter and electromagnetic energy. Subtle energy that cannot be seen or measured fills the other 96% of the universe. And, we can observe the effects of subtle energy on living organisms. Dr. Kronn was involved in experiments with Dr. Yan Xin, a qigong master and medical doctor who could repeatedly affect the half-life of a radioactive substance, americium-24, by projecting subtle energy (chi) to it. Knowing that neither electrical nor magnetic fields can influence the decay rate of radioactive elements, this effect of chi on radioactivity defies explanation. But Dr. Yan Xin's chi did modify the characteristic behavior of matter. Dr. Kronn concludes that chi, subtle energy, belongs to the subatomic world. This subtle energy is a fifth force next to the four known fundamental forces of nature.

In his seminal work, *Vibrational Medicine*, Richard Gerber, MD describes this shift in paradigm. The Einsteinian paradigm as applied to vibrational medicine sees human beings as networks of complex energy fields that interface with physical/cellular systems. Vibrational medicine attempts to interface with these primary subtle energy fields. James Oschmann's book, *Energy Medicine: The Scientific Basis,* covers extensive research providing a scientific basis as to why chemical communication no longer adequately explains the incalculable array of processes occurring in living organisms. He concludes that many processes even supersede our conventional notions of electromagnetic communication. Instead, brilliant research indicates that the mechanisms involved in communications are quantum processes. Research illustrates that these mechanisms involve an array of advanced scientific concepts: quantum coherence as described by Herbert Frölich, spin resonance as described by Mae Wan Ho and Emilio Del Giudice, biophotonic communication as described by Fritz Albert Popp, and the concepts of non-locality, discontinuity, and entanglement in the quantum model of medicine developed by Drouin and Goswami.

Bruce Lipton reinforces the frequency model of communication in his book, *The Biology of Belief*. Lipton calls for a revision in our current understanding that cells receive and process information purely on a chemical basis. Lipton posits that cellular receptors can also read vibrational energy fields such as light, sound, and radio frequencies. If an energy vibration in the environment resonates with a receptor's antenna, it will alter the protein's charge, causing the receptor to change shape. Dr. Herbert Frölich discovered that biomolecules emit and receive electromagnetic as well as vibrational energy. The receiving or sending of energy causes a change in shape, which induces a change in behavior. Frölich provided mathematical models to demonstrate the foundation for the work of Dr. Fritz-Albert Popp, who established that it is light (energy) in the form of biophotons that provides the mode of communication between molecules, cells and DNA.

Perhaps a new model for comprehending the complexity of the energetic communication in the human body can found in the radical ideas proposed by pioneering physicist David Bohm. In 1952, Bohm published his innovative work from Princeton in a paper entitled *Hidden Variables*. This paper introduced his revolutionary theory of *Implicate Order*. Though initially dismissed, this work is finally being reviewed in a more serious light. His research laid the groundwork for a philosophy that underlies the apparent wave-particle behavior of matter. Bohm proposed that underneath the wave particle duality lays a unifying wholeness; that beyond the everyday material world there is a world with a deeper order: the Implicate Order. This implicate order is a subatomic, holographic space of unbroken wholeness. This theory proposes that the behavior of quantum particles are not chance processes. Rather, the motion of particles such as electrons and photons are guided by what he termed underlying pilot waves.

Research is proving that the vacuum of space is anything but empty. The basic structure of the universe is a sea of quantum fields. In this vacuum of space, fluctuations in energy are detectable even in temperatures of absolute zero. And, according to Heisenberg's Uncertainty Principle, particles are in constant motion. Lynn McTaggart investigates these concepts and the cutting-edge scientific research currently being conducted in her book, *The Field*. The so-called vacuum of space - also known as the zero-point state, the source field of infinite potential, or simply 'The Field' - is teeming with quantum potential. In alignment with the philosophy that energy is primary, McTaggart describes human beings, as well as all living things, as a coalescence of energy fields that are connected to everything else in the field. Research indicates that this field is an information source guiding the growth of our minds and bodies. It is this field that must be tapped in order to access our healing.

It seems that science and ancient philosophy arrive at similar conclusions from radically different viewpoints.

> *"From the Great Spirit, came a great unifying force that flowed into things – the flowers of the prairies, blowing wind, rocks, trees, birds, animals – and*

was the same force that had been breathed into the first man. Thus all things were kindred and we were brought together by the same great mystery."
    Luther Standing Bear

"*Tao is whirling emptiness, yet when used it can not be exhausted. Out of this mysterious well flows everything in existence. The ten thousand things are born of being. Being is born of non being.*"
    Lao Tzu

"*The universal substance, ether, is condensed through a movement of molecular polarization, and matter first appears in the gaseous state. From this ether appears four states: understanding and mind, knowledge and life, force and movement, form and resistance.*"   Eliphas Levi

"*Hindu scriptures refer not only to the anu, 'atom', and the paramanu 'beyond on the atom', finer electronic energies, but also to prana 'creative lifetronic force'. Atoms and electrons are blind forces; prana is inherently intelligent".*

Sri Yukteswar

David Bohm believed that within this quantum field of potential energy lay a deeper order, an implicate order. This implicate order is actually a process of continual unfolding, from the implicate order of the quantum field into an explicate order of the material world. That is, the explicate (manifest) order, that which manifests as our observed reality, is the explicate order that unfolds from the underlying implicate (quantum) order. The particle is an abstraction apprehended by our senses. However, this is not a *random* process; as Einstein said, *"God does not play dice with the universe".* The manifest, material world unfolds from and is guided by pilot waves, emerging from the underlying quantum source field. This enfolding and unfolding is the continual dance of creation. And this implicate order unfolds continually with ever increasing complexity.

As Bohm explains, out of the perceived emptiness

particles interact with, respond to, and are informed by an informational potential that allows for manifestation. (Informed by an informational potential will be a key point). This principle functions in the presence of quantum systems, as is illustrated by the double-slit experiment; that is, how the potential manifests as either wave or particle. In other words, as the quantum particle approaches the double slit, it is the *quantum potential* (energy) that organizes the manner in which the trajectory manifests. Quantum forces, "hidden forces", derived from a deeper level of reality, a subatomic world of background energy called the Holomovement, cause the behavior of subatomic particles.

So how is this information useful when discussing health, medicine and the energy body of man? This philosophy of the implicate order can be utilized to help understand healing and the energy body from a radically new perspective. The author would like to propose an innovative approach that could be viewed as a type of quantum blueprint for healing.

In order to discuss this blueprint, a few other

science-based, radical principles essential to this proposal must be introduced. These principles provide a scientific basis from which we can derive this model of a quantum blueprint for health. Allow a space for expansion of the mind as we progress down this path. These radical ideas consider both soliton waves and the mathematical method of the Fourier transform.

First, let us explore soliton waves. In contrast to an electromagnetic wave that dissipates over space and time, a soliton wave is self-reinforcing, maintaining a constant shape and energy as it moves through space and time. It behaves like a particle in that it maintains its shape at a constant speed. Moreover, a soliton wave retains its structure even when it interacts with other soliton waves. As mentioned earlier, the "fifth force" also does not weaken with distance, and penetrates most materials and shielding. For a visual aid, imagine dropping a stone into a still pond. If the wave created from that action could move through the water in perpetuity without losing its shape, this would be analogous to a soliton wave. By contrast, waves within our electromagnetic spectrum dissipate their energy within the resulting medium. To further illustrate, imagine that you could drop two separate stones in that still pond, and their resulting wave patterns could move through one another with out interference, loosing neither shape nor velocity. These principles will be important as we discuss the energy of meridian channels.

Next, consider the Fourier transform, which is a mathematical system useful for exploring quantum mechanics. The Fourier transform models the expression of the sum of converging sine wave functions. In the book *The Holographic Soul*, Mike Hockney explains how Fourier mathematics can model energy wave conversions. He states that the basis of the mechanism of quantum mechanics (and holography) can be found in the Fourier Transform. These mathematical formulas describe the mechanism of conversion of frequency functions from the field of infinite potential into the space-time functions of the material world.

How do these seemingly divergent and radical scientific principles unite to depict a quantum blueprint? And how does this create a working model system that integrates crucial information escaping the current practice of conventional Western medicine? The following is a philosophy for health based on the previously discussed scientific principles.

The totality of man comprises exceedingly intricate and complex, multifaceted chemical, electrical and subtle energy systems. Energy is primary; chemistry is secondary. Physical changes are preceded by changes in the subtle energy systems. With advanced technology, those energy changes can be observed and measured.

In every second we are presented with an infinitesimal amount of data that cannot possibly be processed, compiled or directed solely with chemistry and electricity. Research has proven that communication occurs due to quantum processes and is guided by the interaction of biophotons within DNA. Perhaps the meridians of the subtle body, work in conjunction with DNA to communicate across the entire body instantaneously. The photons could communicate through the use of the body's quantum Internet, the meridian system. Through this, a significant amount of functionality would occur autonomously in the subtle energy body, increasing the speed and functionality of cell maintenance. We can refer to numerous other scientific experiments and clinical evidence to support this hypothesis.

Each acupuncture channel exists as a quantum entity. Each has the potential to exist as both wave and particle. As quantum entities, the meridians communicate with each other and the entire body instantaneously through the quantum principles of non-locality, discontinuity, and entanglement.

The meridians are transducers of information from the field of infinite potential energy to the physical expression of energy. Per David Bohm, out of the perceived emptiness, particles (meridians) interact with, respond to, and are informed by an informational potential that allows for manifestation. The non-anatomical, energetic meridians are implicate and the result of the energy in organs, thinking and emotions is explicate. The particle that manifests is an abstraction finding manifestation through our senses (transducers). Each meridian is a transducer for screening and apprehending information into a manageable state for use in maintaining homeostasis. The electromagnetic field is a hologram constructed from the interference patterns in the individual meridians.

Energy in a meridian may be in the form of a soliton wave. A meridian has the capacity to align with an infinitesimal array of soliton waves from the source field. These soliton waves exist in the quantum field of potential, as pilot waves in the implicate order. The waves within each meridian are self-reinforcing, maintaining a constant shape and energy. They behave like particles in that they maintain shape at a constant speed. And, these waves retain their structure even as they interact with other waves of each individual meridian. These waves are energy in formation, or information. This information manifests as particles as it aligns with the organs and tissues along a specific channel. This energy informs on a multidimensional level, manifesting physical as well as mental, emotional and spiritual states. A belief of many cultural systems of healing is that this information is a type of consciousness.

The standing waves do not transfer the energy. Rather, they interact with the wave function of the meridian, effecting a change in the physical. When this energy is affected via an external source (environmental changes) or an internal source (a change in emotions or conscious thought), the standing wave itself does not change. What changes is an alignment with the new wave function. The moving energy is not electromagnetic energy; rather, it is a standing wave pattern. It is the interaction between standing waves and three-dimensional matter within the meridian system that produces the change in energy. The wave function of the meridian exists as a standing wave, which manifests on the physical plane as the particle. The pilot waves of implicate order are informing the body and the mind on all levels. We are the synthesis of nonlocal and local information, connected to the subatomic level and communicating in a holistic manner. An alignment with a new wave of potential creates change in the energy of the meridian that can be observed prior to any physical change. This change may be instantaneous – non-local and discontinuous. Or conversely, changes may appear slowly over time.

Energy systems interface with subatomic quantum space that integrates information. From that space, different "choices" can be made that can manifest instantaneously - termed a quantum collapse. When the wave of potential collapses, a new manifestation occurs as a changed reality. But here is the rub: thinking will not necessarily make it so. The ultimate challenge will be discovering how to access zero point space to allow for the change. The ancients teach that we must shift the focus internally, where we possess the ultimate power for change. Is this not why the great masters instilled the importance of meditation? This practice places the body in a neutral state where it has access to the field. When we suspend linear, logical thoughts that direct according to past situations, the energy systems of the body engage their innate wisdom for returning to homeostasis. The process cannot be forced, yet we *can* place the body in a neutral state where it can access the field of all potential. In one sense, this places the body in a wave state from which a new particle state can manifest. If we can suspend the deductive reasoning of the active consciousness of the mind and open the inductive subconscious, we open possibilities for a different collapse of the wave function to produce different physical outcomes. Each meridian has its own unique blueprint or archetype. Vital energy through the meridian contains its own wisdom of inductive reasoning based on the physical particle of the cell or tissue, along with what is available in the archetype of the perfect or optimal function.

Moreover, evidence for this theory of a quantum blueprint has been derived from clinical observation. Instantaneous changes in the meridian flow that lead to lasting healing have been observed numerous times in practice. These instantaneous changes are accompanied by an immediate change in conscious awareness. It could be a sudden realization of a new perspective, a release of an emotional or mental block, or surrender to trusting the body's innate healing wisdom. Since the meridians are quantum entities, as the energy (wave function) changes, the particle changes its physical manifestation of expression. In physics, this is known as the quantum collapse of the wave function. The collapse of the wave function manifests as a new particle.

Advanced technology allows for observation and analysis of these changing energy states, providing new possibilities for interventions at much earlier stages in the healing process. ElectroDermal Analysis allows us to observe the energetic state of the meridians. Each meridian has its own field of potential; each has an access point which helps to open a window to the quantum field. Many cultures teach that each meridian is essentially a consciousness center for a wholeness that expresses as either neutrality or a polarity in that channel. As a change in that flow or a change in perspective registers, it can be observed instantaneously as it registers change in the meridian. Energy disruptions that indicate out of phase alignment or energy impedances can be caught and monitored before physical tissue change occurs. As the subtle energy, or consciousness, changes alignment to a new pilot wave from the implicate order, its expression is manifested as a change within the explicate order. The consciousness of that particular energy center manifests an instantaneous change that affects material, linear reality with a different expression. The progressively positive changes in energy states that build health can be observed. Understanding the energetic intelligence of the body, we have a manner to access the energetic environment and can take steps to modify outcomes.

Meridians, subtle energy systems and electromagnetic fields comprise a network of parallel processes in one realm, while chemistry is a linear step-by-step process in another. Each has its vital importance to the maintenance, growth and evolution of the organism. Our human system is connected to the frequency domain outside of the space and time of the three-dimensional world through our subtle energy body. The organs within the meridians are transducers for the information specific to that system. What is perceived as the transformation of the wave function into the particle (referred to as the collapse of the wave function), which results in a different material expression, may be beyond merely an electromagnetic transfer of energy. A change in material expression represents a change in a specific wave function, and how the body is experiencing its interface with that wave function. Either the standing wave is life affirming - resulting in growth and maintenance - or imbalanced, where we experience pain and discomfort. This imbalance provides an experience, and yes, even a road map from which we can learn to take steps to align with a wave function that sustains and promotes vibrant health.

As mentioned earlier, mathematical formulas exist that theoretically describe the mechanism of conversion of frequency functions from the field of infinite potential into the space-time functions of the material world. It has been proposed that the mind, via Fourier transform, can convert frequency functions of the subatomic world into space-time functions of the 3-D material realm. From this line of logic we could infer that the meridians, via Fourier transform, can convert frequency functions of the subatomic (implicate) world into our three-dimensional one. Likewise, through inverse Fourier transform, humanity possesses the capacity to enfold its explicate experience back into the field of infinite potential in a continual evolving dance of creation. We have yet to discover the immense depth of our true human potential.

Let us take a look at some clinical evidence that supports and illustrates the working of this hypothesis.

Not long after completing my internship at the Institute of Natural Health Sciences, I received a call to consult with a colleague on a case. She was working with a man we will call John, who had a cancerous tumor in his chest. He was scheduled for a procedure the following day to locate and mark the area intended for radiation. My colleague was contemplating giving John a remedy that was homeopathic to his physical, mental and emotional symptoms. John was seeking alternative medicine in addition to his scheduled radiation therapy. He was open to trying a homeopathic remedy that could have a positive effect on his healing, even if only to augment his conventional therapy. His medical doctors saw no harm in trying the tiny white "sugar pills". John wanted to be in the best frame of mind and body for his upcoming treatments. He had, also, been carrying an enormous burden for years, struggling with the loss of someone very dear to him. The remedy that was proposed seemed to be an excellent choice. I had seen the same remedy make remarkable shifts in emotional healing from deep grief in my own practice. My colleague asked for my prayers to help positively influence his healing.

The next morning, his physicians were dumbfounded. The technician was unable to locate the presence of any tumor in the area that was targeted for treatment. Several tests were done to reconfirm this finding; even expanding the search area to ensure something else had not been missed. John never had that surgery. Neither did he require radiation, nor chemotherapy. He just smiled and said his miracle just meant, "It's not my time to go. I must have more work to do."

Now, I want to be perfectly clear here. This does *not* in any way imply that homeopathy should be used to treat cancer, or that it cures cancer. Likewise, it does not imply that homeopathy should be employed in place of conventional therapies for cancer. This case is presented to illustrate a number of points.

First, experiences such as these fall outside our understanding of healing in the material, linear model. But what happens in these cases of "spontaneous remission" where it appears an instantaneous healing has occurred?

Perhaps the perspective of a blueprint that operates within the realm of quantum physics may shed a different light on the issue. We have presented the idea of a quantum collapse. As energy systems interface with subatomic space, different "choices" can be made that can manifest instantaneously. When the wave of potential collapses, a new manifestation occurs as a changed reality. However, the "choice" is not of necessity a conscious choice. Change can be occurring in the subconscious mind that underlies our level of conscious awareness. This is already known from the study of trauma. In John's case, a changing set of thought patterns, emotions, and beliefs all converged simultaneously, merging to produce a shift that resulted in a quantum collapse and emergence of the new reality. This change in perceived reality now manifests as a different energy stream to the whole human instrument. It is like changing the channel on the television and seeing something new. And this process does not apply solely to the big healings like cancer. It can be small changes that shift our perspective, directing us down a new path where things change to support our highest good.

Second, we of course have to address the notion of

the placebo effect. That is, a certain percentage of people experience positive results because their expectation of healing somehow affects the body's own chemistry. Maybe this view is slightly skewed. Perhaps a certain percentage responds favorably not because they believe it will work better, but because they have no false conceptions that it will not work. Their minds are not aligned with the story that it cannot work, or the tale of how many other things have to be possible in order for it to work. In any case, it would be a bit of a stretch to attribute the sudden disappearance of a cell mass to the placebo effect.

Another client, Susan, scheduled an initial consultation to address menopausal issues. Susan was a diabetic. Her EAV readings revealed a consistent energy impedance in the Liver meridian. This situation persisted for several months despite several remedies and supplements. At one appointment, she was visibly more agitated than in the past. She had recently visited her father, with whom she had a contentious relationship most of her life. She began to relay the story of the encounter. It just so happened that I was testing her Liver meridian at that point when she asked me, "Do you think all this anger

I have toward my father has anything to do with my diabetes?" I asked her to explore that a bit further. As she was unraveling the story, she seemed to have a sudden realization and shift in consciousness. At that same point, the impedance within her Liver meridian released, and her readings balanced. This was a rare moment of serendipity, a gift to be able to witness. That experience presented an opportunity to understand subtle energy body from an entirely new perspective. Susan's sudden shift in consciousness was accompanied by a profound shift in the subtle energy body. Even more profound, her insulin requirements were reduced by half from that day forward. There was no drug, remedy, nor supplement involved. But the sudden realization, the quantum collapse, had a profound effect on the physical body. Susan was still a diabetic, and still required insulin, however, her financial burden had been substantially reduced.

Both John and Susan were amazing teachers. Their healing journeys opened a door, for me, to a deeper understanding of our internal healing power. These experiences led my clinical research down a truly innovative path. Usually, the approach in scientific research is to propose a theory, then conduct an experiment to prove that theory. Of course, this by definition implies bias. And, this bias is an even more valid point since the Double Slit experiment proved that the outcome is determined by how the procedure is observed. However, in these cases it was the opposite. I had clinical observations that defied conventional explanation, then had to search for theories to explain those observations. More information detailing the results of this research can be found in *The Power of Vibrational Medicine: Healing with the Bioacoustics of Nature.*

Communication within living organisms can no longer be adequately explained through strictly chemical or mechanical means, nor through a myopic view into the material realm to the exclusion of the energetic realm. Every organ, tissue and cell has its own resonant frequency, which when operating efficiently, resonate and work harmoniously together. When this frequency is altered, loss of coherence ensues that can lead to disease. Changes that affect the healing process can be detected on an energetic level prior to physical manifestation, yet these energetic changes remain undetected by conventional diagnostics. By ignoring the energy body, information crucial to the healing process is being missed in our current practice of conventional Western medicine. Knowing that illness is initiated by imbalances in the energy systems of the body, methods to detect and to correct these imbalances must be integral for a comprehensive health system.

CHAPTER 10

CLOSING

"The greatest illusion of this world is the illusion of separation. Things you think are separate and different are actually one and the same. We are all one people, but we live as if divided. "   Guru Pathik

Out there...

We want to dispel darkness, rid our world of the things that bind, hurt and tear at people. We turn our collective backs on the suffering of humanity, convinced that the darkness is somewhere "out there". It exists in a different town or in a different country, and it doesn't affect us - until it does. And then we stand dumbfounded as to how this could have happened. But, the darkness is not "out there", vilified in exterior demons that are waiting to attack. If we want to dispel the darkness, we have to turn around, each of us, and face that which is within.

First, we must acknowledge the existence of darkness within each of us, instead of projecting out onto other neighbors and eventually, other countries. Other countries are ultimately made of people. As long as we project outward and see everything as outside of ourselves we feel safe and vindicated. But the illusion of outward pushes us farther apart as a human family, and farther from a place of healing. Each of us has the innate capacity to nurture as well as to kill to protect our loved ones. Denying our basic instincts of survival or our baser, animal nature robs us of tremendous power. It is in these instincts, where we know our environment through the gift of our five senses, which provides the richness of our existence and the power to thrive. And in our base natures the law of polarity exists, where the best of nature lives with the worst.

We have seen that when great tragedies strike the nation, divisions dissolve and we unite in our common humanity. We bear witness to the depths of which humanity sinks to commit such atrocities against human life. Yet, this is often paralleled by the heights to which we can soar when we pull together as a human family, to extend compassion and strength to aid those who are wounded and suffering.

In the single horrendous act of dropping the twin towers on September 11, 2001, we witnessed the demonstration of extreme polarities and capabilities of mankind. We witnessed the depth of depravity to which humans could sink. Yet in the wake of this tragedy we also witnessed the heights to which humanity could ascend. Through our common humanity and our innate desire to connect and protect, we all united through kindness, generosity, love and compassion. From the wisdom gained from this experience, each of us can turn to our own horrific wounds that are the price of experiencing life. And that same life experience is also the source of the ecstasy that fills the heart.

This propensity for the depths and the heights exists within each and every one of us. Yet denial of that fact is the root of much suffering. We have been convinced that certain feelings and emotions are bad and should be suppressed; that feeling anxious, sad or even angry is wrong and indicates that we may have some sort of disorder (and yes, we have a drug for that). If we are taught that our bodies and mind are weak, that we are victims of our environment, we tend to give up hope. This undermines and even reverses our extraordinary capacity to positively affect our own healing processes.

There is clear evidence to support the fact that symptoms do not necessarily indicate that something is broken, or that we are incapable of repair without outside intervention. Rather, symptoms can be read as a roadmap indicating an imbalance; nature's way of alerting our conscious mind that a deficiency or excess needs to be addressed. When we change how we view our symptoms and learn what information they are trying to convey, we change our relationship to them. We can learn to read the language of our inner wisdom when we consider symptoms as a roadmap to healing. When the energy that originally formed the malfunction is removed or changed, there is nothing from which this manifestation will continue to form. Changing the wave changes the particle. A change in consciousness that is aligned with a different potential or possibility creates different reality outcomes – changes the quantum collapse. Expanding on this philosophy, we can read distress, degradation, unrest and even violence in society and our natural environment as indicators of tremendous imbalances where intervention and assistance are most needed.

Consciousness is the substance of form, and forms are created based on past conditioning registered in the brain, mind and heart. When we change our energetic resonance and our conscious alignments, different outcomes are established. Our energy systems continuously interface with subatomic quantum space (the field of infinite potential). From that space of infinite potential, different choices can be made that manifest instantaneously in a new quantum collapse. As we change the waveform, instantaneous and discontinuously the particle also changes, following its dual nature. This can instantaneously manifest a changed reality. When beliefs no longer serve our highest intent (and positive evolution of the consciousness of our collective), dissonance ensues, which will produce discomfort. This discomfort will persist until the pain of the stagnant form outweighs the pain of growth. The armor of energy required to maintain the defenses around the wound could be better utilized to effect massive healing.

This energy is real energy. It can be utilized in numerous life-supporting ways. It is time to break free from the trance of the material realm. The five senses are only one part of the vast picture of our multidimensional experience. The focus on the particle to the exclusion of the wave tends to dis-integrate us from our natural environment. A static tissue sample in a test tube or petri dish is disconnected from the dynamics present in a whole living organism. The study of the wave portion of life engages the energetic relationship of the whole organism and the organism's integration with its environment.

This work provides evidence that our conventional medical approach speaks to only a fraction of the truth. It calls for expansive research into the energy nature of man that contains immense information that we have yet to apprehend or understand. These energy systems contain valuable insight regarding the roadblocks preventing the embodiment of our full, vibrant, unstoppable potential for growth and healing. This is not a suggestion to spring open the soul cages all at once and run wild. But I have witnessed profound change happen in an instant with the recognition of one piece of missing information that changes an entire life. Because of the lessons learned, the knowledge assimilated and understood becomes a wisdom that is not learned any other way. It is a bodily, experiential wisdom learned on all levels, felt on all senses, embraced by body, mind and spirit.

A simple act of kindness - a few warm words, a helping, and gentle touch - contains the power to instantaneously change a moment, an attitude and possibly the trajectory of a life. In this, we find our common humanity and our connection to the forces of life. Without this positive connection and building of community, life force contracts, isolates, becomes small and withdraws. Without it community and health diminish, sometimes even to the point of death.

I have seen enough miracles to know that healing happens. When you have your health, you really do have everything.

And if there is a will, we will find a way, perhaps a different way, a better way, with new tools and a quantum leap in perception. We can then use this valuable information to direct our extraordinary, unlimited potential as human beings. We can positively influence our evolution, healing and spiritual growth to achieve the best life possible for ourselves, and by extension our community and our world. And…ultimately, love wins - even though it may not appear to in every instance, but enough to make the journey on this little blue planet worth the trip as we remember our connection to the whole, each of us comprising at once both wings of light and feet of clay.

BIBLIOGRAPHY

Abu-Asab, Ph.D., M., Amri, Ph.D., H., & Micozzi, M.D., Ph.D., M. S. (2013). *Avicenna's Medicine: A New Translation of the 11th Century Cannon with Practical Applications for Integrative Health Care.* Rochester, VT: Healing Arts press.

Ahlbom, A., Bridges, J., & Mattsson, M. (2007, March 21). Possible Effects of EMF on Human Health. *Scientific Committee on Emerging and Newly Identified Health Risks (SCENIHR)*, 3 - 63. Retrieved from https://ec.europa.eu/health/ph_risk/committees/04_s cenihr/docs/scenihr_o_007.pdf

Beinfield, H., & Korngold, E. (1991). *Between Heaven and Earth: A Guide to Chinese Medicine.* New York, NY: Ballantine Publishing Group.

Bioinformative Medicine. (2010). Retrieved from http://www.magnetotherapy.de/fileadmin/download s/pdfs/E/AMS_Info_Ausland_part_I_to_III_englisc h_with_pictures.pdf

Childre, D., Martin, H., & Beech, D. (1999). *The HeartMath Solution.* New York, NY: HarperCollins Publishers.

Chronic Disease Prevention and Health Promotion. (2017). Retrieved from https://www.cdc.gov/chronicdisease/about/preventi on.htm

Dechar, Lorie Eve. (2006). *Five Spirts: Alchemical Acupuncture for Psychological and Spiritual Healing.* New York, NY: Lantern Books

Drouin, P. (2014). *Creative Integrative Medicine: A Medical Doctor's Journey toward a New Vision for Health Care.* Bloomington, IN: Balboa Press.

Eanes, R. (2004). EAV Discussions: Electro-Acupuncture Testing, Electro-Acupuncture According to Dr. Voll. Retrieved from http://eavresource.com/wp-content/uploads/2015/02/EAV-Electro-Acupuncture-Testing-Electro-Acupuncture-According-to-Dr.-Voll.pdf

Edwards, S. (2001). Frequency as an Intrinsic Healing Factor. Retrieved from http://www.soundhealthoptions.com/frequency-as-intrinsic-healing-modality

emWave Pro Plus Assessments. (2016). In *Overview - Assessments.* HeartMath: HeartMath Institute.

Ericcson, A. D., Pittaway, K., & Lai, R. (2003). ElectroDermal Analysis, a Scientific Correlation with Pathophysiology. *Explore!* Retrieved from http://eavresource.com/wp-content/uploads/2015/02/Electro-Dermal-Analysis-study-final-proof.pdf

F., L. M., Tsuei, J. J., & Zhao, Z. (1990). Study of the bioenergetic measurement of acupuncture points for determination of correct dosages of allopathic or homeopathic medicines in the treatment of diabetes mellitus. *American Journal of Acupuncture, 18*).

Gerber, M.D., R. (1998). (1996) *Vibrational Medicine: New Choices for Healing Ourselves*. Santa Fe, NM: Bear & Company.

Goswami, Ph.D., A. (2004). *The Quantum Doctor: A Physicist's Guide to Health and Healing*. Charlottesville, VA: Hampton Roads Publishing.

Goswami, Ph.D., A., Reed, R. E., & Goswami, M. (1993). *The Self-Aware Universe: How Consciousness Creates the Material World*. New York, NY: Penguin Putnam, Inc.

Grigorova, Ph.D., N. G. (2012). *Electro Acupuncture by Voll (EAV) and Homeopathy*. Santa Clara, CA: Milkanan Publishing.

Hahnemann, S. (1982). *Organon of Medicine* (6th Ed.). Blaine, Washington: Cooper Publishing.

Hammer, Leon, M.D. (1990) *Dragon Rises, Red Bird Flies*. Barrytown, New York: Station Hill Press

Heart, Bear. (1996) *The Wind is My Mother, The Life and Teaching of a Native American Shaman*. New York, NY: The Berkley Publishing Group

Heart Rate Variability Overview. (2017). Retrieved from www.heartmath.com

Ho, M. (2008). *The Rainbow and the Worm: The Physics of Organisms* (3rd Ed.). Hackensack, NJ: World Scientific Publishing Co. Pte. Ltd.

Imagine Films. (2021) *Infinite Potential: The Life and Ideas of David Bohm*. Dublin, Ireland: Imagine Films

Kalyuzhny, G. (Volume 4 Number 121, September 2016). The Influence of Electromagnetic Pollution on Living Organisms: Historical Trends and Forecasting Changes. Retrieved from http://www.energytoolsint.com/

Kaptchuk, T. J. (2000). *The Web That Has No Weaver: Understanding Chinese Medicine*. New York, NY: McGraw-Hill Publshing.

Laszlo, E. (2077) (2007). *Science and the Akashic Field; An Integral Theory of Everything* (2nd ed.). Rochester, VT: Inner Traditions .

Leonhardt, H. (1980). *Fundamentals of Electroacupuncture According to Voll*. C. Beckers Buchdruckerei, Uelzen: Medizinisch Literarische Verlagsgesellschaft mbH.

Levi, Eliphas. (2000). *The Mysteries of the Qabala*. York Beach, Maine: Samuel Weiser.

Lipton, Ph.D., B. H. (2005). *The Biology of Belief: Unleashing the Power of Unconsciousness, Matter & Miracles*. Santa Rosa, CA: Mountain of Love / Elite Books.

Madill, P. (1979, December). Electroacupuncture: A true and legitimate preventative medicine. *American Journal of Acupuncture.*

Maman, F., & Unsoeld, T. (2016). *The Tao of Sound: Acoustic Healing for the 21st Century* (Second ed.). Malibu, CA: Tama-Do, The Academy of Sound, Color and Movement.

McCraty, Ph.D., R. (2015). *Science of the Heart: Exploring The Role of the Heart in Human Performance, Volume 2*. Boulder Creek, CA: HeartMath Institute.

McCraty, R., Barrios-Choplin, B., Rozman, D., Atkinson, M., & Watkins, A. D. (1998). The impact of a new emotional self-management program on stress, emotions, heart rate variability, DHEA and cortisol. *Integrative Physiological and Behavioral Science, 33*(2), 151-70. Retrieved from https://www.ncbi.nlm.nih.gov/pubmed/9737736

McTaggart, L. (2002). *The Field; The Quest for the Secret Force of the Universe*. New York, NY: HarperCollins Publishers.

Oschman, J. L. (2016). *Energy Medicine: The Scientific Basis* (Second ed.). Dover, New Hampshire: Elsevier Ltd.

Oschman, Ph.D, J. L. (2002). *Energy Medicine: The Scientific Basis*. Edinburgh, UK: Elsevier Sciences Limited.

Pischinger, Alfred (2007). *The Extracellular Matrix and Ground Regulation: Basis for Holistic Biological Medicine*. Berkley, CA: North Atlantic Books

Pittaway, K. S. (2002). *Electro Dermal Analysis: Student Handbook*. Livonia, MI: Institute of Natural Health Science.

Pittaway, N.D., Ph.D., K. S. (2001). *Electro Dermal Screening: Student Handbook*. Livonia, MI: Institute of Natural Health Sciences.

Rosch, M.D., P. J. (2015). 2014 (Amazon shows 2014 for 2nd ed.) *Bioelectromagnetic and Subtle Energy Medicine* (2nd ed.). Boca Raton, FL: CRC Press.

Rubik, B. (2002, December). The biofield hypothesis: its biophysical basis and role in medicine. *Journal of Alternative and Complimentary Medicine, 8,* 703-717. http://dx.doi.org/https://dx.doi.org/10.1089/10755530260511711

Rubik, Ph.D., B., Muehsan, Ph.D., D., Hammerschlag, Ph.D., R., & Jain Ph.D., S. (2015). Biofield Science and Healing: History, Terminology and Concepts. Retrieved from https://www.ncbi.nlm.nih.gov/pmc/articles/PMC4654789/, Biofield Science and Healing: History, Terminology, and Concepts

Swanson, Ph.D., C. V. (2010). *Life Force: The Scientific Basis: Breakthrough Physics of Energy Medicine, Healing, Chi and Quantum Consciousness, Volume II*. Tucson, AZ: Poseidia Press.

Thayer, J. F., Yamamoto, S. S., & Brosschot, J. F. (2010, May 28, 2010). The relationship of autonomic imbalance, heart rate variability and cardiovascular risk factors. *International Journal of Cardiology,*

141(2), 122-131. Retrieved from www.internationaljournal of cardiology.com/article/S0167-5273(09)01487-91/fulltext

Tsuei, J. (1996, May/June). Bio-Energetic Medicine: Scientific Evidence in Support of Acupuncture and Meridian Theory, Part II, The Past, Present and Future of EDSS. *Engineering in Medicine and Biology, Volume 15, Number 3).*

Tsuji, H., Larson, M. G., Venditti, F. J., Manders, E. S., Evans, J. C., Feldman, C. L., & Levy, D. (1996, December 1st). Impact of Reduced Heart Rate Variability on Risk for Cardiac Events. *Circulation, 94*, 2850-2855.

Tzu, Lao. (1995). *The Tao Te Ching of Lao Tzu.* New York, NY: St. Martin's Press

Voll, R. (1980). The Phenomena of medicine testing in electroacupuncture according to Voll. *American Journal of Acupuncture,* 8).

Wijk, R. V. (2014). *Light in Shaping Life: Biophotons in Biology and Medicine.* Meluna, Geldermalsen, The Netherlands: Ten Brink B.V., Meppel, The Netherlands.

Yogananda, Paramanhansa. (1998 Thirteenth ed.) *The Autobiography of a Yogi.* Los Angeles, CA: The Self-Realization Fellowship.

ABOUT THE AUTHOR

Gretchen Weger Snell, PhD, DNM, is a clinician, instructor and researcher in the field of natural and energy medicine. She utilizes traditional healing methods in combination with the latest technological advances in the field of alternative and natural healthcare to teach clients to build health naturally. In addition, Dr. Snell is an instructor and faculty member at the Institute of Natural Health Sciences in Farmington Michigan. Her research has been published in:

The Power of Vibrational Medicine: Healing with the Bioacoustics of Nature
(Gretchen Weger Snell, PhD, 2019)

For more information, visit:
http://www.naturalpathconsulting.com

Made in the USA
Monee, IL
27 May 2021